Dimensions of Radionics
Techniques of Instrumented Distant-Healing
A Manual of Radionic Theory and Practice

by
David V. Tansley, D.C.

in collaboration with
Malcolm Rae
and Aubrey T. Westlake,
B.A., M.B., B.Chir., M.R.C.S., L.R.C.P.

Brotherhood of Life, Inc.
Albuquerque, New Mexico

David V. Tansley 1934 – 1988

Printing History

DIMENSIONS OF RADIONICS

©David V. Tansley 1977
First Published in the U.K. by
The C.W. Daniel Company Ltd., Saffron Walden, 1977
First American edition published by
Brotherhood of Life Publishing 1992, reprinted 1997

ISBN 0-914732-29-3

Brotherhood of Life Publishing
110 Dartmouth, SE
Albuquerque, NM 87106 USA
Internet: http://www.brotherhoodoflife.com

Printed in the United States of America

ACKNOWLEDGEMENTS

Theosophical Publishing House: *The Mystery of Healing. The Astral Body* by A.E. Powell. Theosophical University Press: *The Secret Doctrine* by H.P. Blavatsky. The Lucis Press: *A Treatise on Cosmic Fire, Esoteric Healing and A Treatise on White Magic* by Alice A. Bailey, and *The Soul — The Quality of Life.* Wildwood House: *Experiments in Distant Influence* by L. L. Vasiliev. Ganesh & Co: *The Serpent Power* by Sir John Woodroffe. Rider & Co: *Man the Measure of All Things* by Sri Krishna Prem & Sri Madhava Ashish. Turnstone Press: *Dowsing* by Tom Graves. Edgar Cayce Foundation: *Chiropractic Reference Notebook.* Routledge Kegan & Paul: *The I Ching* translated by Richard Wilhelm. *Main Currents in Modern Thought: Compute and Evolve* by Jose Arquelles. Abelard: *The Intelligent Universe* by David Foster. Hahnemann Publishing Society: *The Organon of Medicine* by Samuel Hahnemann. C.W. Daniel Co. Ltd: *Heal Thyself* by Dr. Edward Bach. Cooperative Publishing Co: *The Unseen Link* by Ethel Belle Morrow. University of California Press: *The Yellow Emperor's Classic of Internal Medicine* by I. Veith. L.N. Fowler & Co. Ltd: *The Vital Body* by Max Heindel. Academy of Parapsychology and Medicine: *How to make use of the Field of Mind Theory* by Dr. Elmer Green. Rudolf Steiner Publishing Co: *Spiritual Science and Medicine* by Rudolph Steiner. H.K. Lewis & Co. Ltd: *Colour and Cancer* by Dr. C.E. Iredell. University Books. *The Odic Force* by Karl Von Reichenbach. Marshall McLuhan Newsletter.

My special thanks to Richard A. Belsham for the excellent line drawings of the Magneto-Geometric Radionic Analyser, the Potency Simulators and the Potency Preparer.

I feel that this is one of the most important books on radiesthesia and
radionics since Abbé Mermet's *Principles and Practice of Radionics.*
Certainly it is one of the clearest accounts of the subject that I have
ever read – a brilliant piece of work and beautifully written. I believe it
will become a standard classic in its field.

Colin Wilson, 1977

CONTENTS

LIST OF ILLUSTRATIONS

FOREWORD

In his earlier book 'Radionics and The Subtle Anatomy of Man' the author pointed out a suggestible relationship as between Theosophical ideas coming from the East and the art of Radionics which is essentially Western. I understand that he was led to such a suggestibility in order to ensure that Radionics did not become too materialistic in terms of electro-magnetism, and gave a balancing credence to those lighter vibrations which we know as spirit and thought. But in his other book 'Radionics — Interface with The Ether Fields' he also noted what may prove perhaps to be a more important relationship as between Radionics and modern molecular biology, and where it is established that matter is interfaced with thought in the triple codons and words of the DNA. One suspects that in due course the facts of molecular biology will respectfully supercede the Theosophical ideas so that the study of the etheric will come to be based almost wholly on Western science and art.

It appears that my recent book 'The Intelligent Universe' may have added some strength to the contribution of science in explaining the etheric realms. What I discovered over thirty years of study was that the basis of the universe is data and intelligence, and that such psychic categories must replace our former treatment of the universe as a structure of energy. I was not the originator of such ideas which go back to the Cambridge School of the 1930's and associated with such famous names as Sir Arthur Eddington and Sir James Jeans. Indeed, my own attention was focussed on the matter when Sir Arthur Eddington stated that "We suspect that the stuff of the world is mind-stuff." This is the proposition which I have explored and found reinforced by modern science by two new factors: In the first place the structure of matter is very similar to the digitised structure of electronic computers, and secondly, that the source of organic life in the DNA molecule operates through 'words' which have a specific triple code comparable to the binary code used in computers. Thus we may now reasonably accept the saying of St. John that "In the beginning was the Word."

This is the field being explored by the techniques of Radionics and this book is an important review of the art as it exists at present. Radionics is still in the early exploratory stage as the author makes clear and must contain fallacies as well as truths but this compromise it shares with formal science. Formal science also explores the occult although it may do so with expensive linear accelerators revealing such bizzarrities as Quarks and Charm.

However, Radionics differs from formal science in one important respect in that a human operator is indispensible although he may be aided by material devices. As the author points out this fact makes special demands on those who investigate or practice the subject since it calls for a high degree of inner mental and emotional discipline in order to secure signals of a high signal-to-noise ratio. As I see it, this means that those who practice this subject have to develop a very sensitive and artistic state of mind for they are exploring territory 'Where Angels fear to tread.'

The subject has its analogy in music where a violinist has his violin which is a mere instrument. But somehow that violinist has the ability to produce sweet music which is not inherent in the violin itself. Thus I think we should talk about the *Art* of Radionics as we talk about the Art of Medicine and realising that an important and inescapable facet is the nature of the human being who is involved and the degree to which he himself can manifest higher psychic qualities such as inner quiet, the power of sustained attention and emotional sensibility. All are basic necessities for an artist.

Over the next hundred years it is certain that Man will recast his views of reality and that the strange nature of the occult and the etheric will be established beyond doubt. I would also be certain that the major breakthrough will come from molecular biology. Radionics is particularly oriented towards the healing of the human body and the master programmes which control the normal health of the human body are in the codes of our DNA. Thus, as the author has suggested, I see the next stage of development of Radionics merging with molecular biology since both are based on 'the power of the word' which is the basis of thought. I find it significant that in the method used by the healing Radionic practitioner he needs to have a 'witness' such as a drop of blood or a hair from the person being treated. But the central feature of such a drop of blood or hair is the DNA therein centrally embedded and which knows everything about every health function of the human body. Every single molecule of our DNA contains the total blueprint for our whole physical existence and I consider that this is the basic reason why Radionics works. Molecular biology has already fully identified the 'receiving set' for the omniscient messages of Cosmic Mind as applied to living creatures . . . it is the DNA without a shadow of a doubt.

I commend this book to all readers searching for reality beyond everyday mere physical self-survival.

David Foster, M.Sc., Ph.D., F.I.E.E., F.I.Mech.E.

— FOREWORD —
TO THE 1992 EDITION

This being the Kali Yuga, a time of dense materialism, voices that speak to the spirit of life are rare, and therefore greatly appreciated. Consider the words of Dr. Edward Bach, discoverer of the flower essence system of healing, regarding dis-ease: "Disease is a kind of consolidation of a mental attitude", meaning *thought,* an unseen force, becomes visible through the physical body. Or the words of Dr. Randolph Stone, visionary founder of the school of polarity therapy concerning pain: "Ninety percent of pain is emotional. Imagination is our worst enemy. There is a spasm in the emotional field before the spasm in the spine and body", meaning *feeling,* an unseen force, penetrates the physical body. Radionics focuses upon the unseen forces that cause disease and utilizes nature's subtle energies for healing.

Dimensions of Radionics contains the writings of souls kindred with the spirit of life. Dr. Tansley offers a detailed overview of the constitution of human energies. His expert, abundant and insightful writings concerning human subtle anatomy and radionic inquiry offers insight, ideas and vistas to all interested in the cause of disease. It takes courage to break from the chains of material thinking. "The mind creates multiplicity everywhere to cover the simplicity in nature," according to Randolph Stone. The ideas presented here are an unfolding toward a deeper understanding of the simplicity of nature.

Section Two details Malcolm Rae's radionic inquiry. In harmony with nature's simplicity, his method remains the zenith of present radionic systems: a method based on the timeless principles of Samuel Hahnemann, combined with the language of nature's intertwined geometric patterns and magnetic force.

What a gift Mr. Rae left us! If one desires a simple, direct method of assessing the pattern of life's energies, digest this book and turn it into practice. For those who are dedicated and willing to work persistently toward proficiency, the method of radionics presented here will surpass all of your expectations. If this book stirs the heart of even a few to delve into the brilliance of Rae's system, combined with the interpretation of subtle energies as described by Dr. Tansley, much suffering, by the graces of nature, will be relieved.

I am indebted to these two souls, David Tansley and Malcolm Rae, for their tireless efforts in seeking higher vibrations for a humanity living in the clutches of the Kali Yuga. Their work and efforts continue through the hearts and hands of others.

ROBERT STEVENS, N.D., N.T.S.
COFOUNDER NEW MEXICO SCHOOL OF NATURAL THERAPEUTICS
ALBUQUERQUE, NEW MEXICO
APRIL, 1992

Preamble

It is with a deep sense of satisfaction that I write a preamble to this important book. For it deals with aspects of a fundamental modern development – the art and science of Radiesthesia.

This development has come from two main sources, which are pursuing their separate ways, perhaps necessarily. But as they both employ the same faculty in and for their findings – the Radiesthetic Faculty – they obviously have much in common.

The first comes from the research work of Dr. Albert Abrams and Ruth Drown in America, and later de la Warr in England, which we now know as Radionics; the second from the medical dowsing activities of French priests and other workers at the beginning of this century. This was taken up in England by Dr. Guyon Richards and his remarkable group of medical doctors who together explored this new form of diagnosis and treatment in their Medical Society for the Study of Radiesthesia. Later this has blossomed into what is called Psionic Medicine under the inspiration of Dr. George Laurence, and has been written up comprehensively by J.H. Reyner under the title of Psionic Medicine — the study and treatment of the causative factors in illness.

A similar coverage is now being done for radionics in this present volume, Dimensions of Radionics. I have known Malcolm Rae and David Tansley for a number of years, and indeed I have been partly responsible for introducing them to this fascinating field of research. Each has approached and developed it in his own way, from very different backgrounds, and at first they did not appreciate how complimentary they were to each other; but when in due course this was realized the result is this fine combined achievement.

David Tansley, after qualifying in Chiropractic in America, came to England to start a practice here. I first met him when, after reading my book *The Pattern of Health*, he asked whether he could meet me with a view to knowing more about radiesthesia and its practical application to healing. He felt, quite correctly, it might be a most valuable adjunct to his chiropractic work. The meeting duly took place and he became enthusiastic about the possibilities which were opened up.

Although a doctor of Chiropractic, he was not medically qualified, and so I suggested he join the Radionic Association to study the subject, rather than the Medical Society for the Study of Radiesthesia, which latter only accepted qualified medical doctors as members.

From this beginning he has gone from strength to strength, and has become one of the outstanding exponents of Radionics; for he has brought to it his training in the occult schools of thought, especially that of Alice Bailey. By so doing he has enlarged and enriched the whole subject, not only in basic concepts but in practical application.

All this he has recorded in his two previous books — *Radionics and the Subtle Anatomy of Man*, and *Radionics-Interface with the Ether Fields*. And now in the third book of the trilogy, in fecund conjunction with Malcolm Rae, there has been added a still wider sweep both in concept and down-to-earth practicality in the present book Dimensions of Radionics.

Malcolm Rae came to this work from a background of a business man with a wide experience in many different commercial undertakings, curiously not really a background which one would have expected to be the best preparation for his present unique research work, which is yielding such rich rewards for fundamental healing. But one should never underestimate the workings of Providence.

Our first contact was in an appraisal of the healing patterns described in *The Pattern of Health* – as to whether there might better and more effective ones. Out of the investigation we made, there developed in due course his remarkable discovery that it was possible, radiesthetically, to find the archetypal pattern of any substance. Also in due course he developed improved designs of the classical radionic diagnostic and treatment instruments. However with further research he abandoned this line of enquiry in favour of an instrument which will enable the archetypal patterns to be used in various ways and particularly in homoeopathic potency preparation by magnetically energized geometric patterns in what he called a Potency Simulator; and subsequently the Rae Magneto-Geometric Radionic Analyser – a truly remarkable creation.

But Malcolm Rae has also suggested tentative explanations, which as far as I know no one else has done, as to how his radionic instruments, together with the geometric patterns, function particularly in the preparation of potencies of homoeopathic remedies. This would appear to be a real advance in basic knowledge.

One may perhaps sum up this combined contribution as an entirely new way of providing 'information' on all levels, so that man is enabled to become whole, and maintain his being in a state of dynamic balance.

All in all there is opening up an exciting and very relevant field of study and research, and so this book is both pertinent and timely. For it is becoming clear that what it deals with, both theoretically and practically, is very necessary, if we, in these disintegrating times, are to find our way out of the materialistic morass into which man is sinking.

But while there is a menace, there is also a challenge and a hope. Are we capable of achieving a rise in our level of consciousness, so that we can gain access to realms of supersensible knowledge and wisdom and act accordingly? The present situation calls, not for more material knowledge, but for a new dimension in thought and awareness — In a word — to a Spiritual Science, to the beginnings of which this book will now add its dedicated contribution.

Aubrey T. Westlake,
B.A., M.B., B.Chir.(Cantab), M.R.C.S., L.R.C.P.
Godshill, Hampshire.
March 1977.

SECTION ONE

Some Fundamental Principles

*General principles are not the less true or important
because from their nature they elude immediate observation; they are like the air, which is not the less
necessary because we neither see nor feel it.*
William Hazlitt

CHAPTER ONE

Towards the Essential Simplicity

The ability to simplify means to eliminate the un-
necessary so that the necessary may speak.
Search for the Real Hans Hofmann

During the last decade or so it has become evident that there is an increasing interest in radionics amongst medical doctors, chiropractors, osteopaths, and others such as masseurs and physiotherapists who are employed full-time as health care professionals. In most instances this interest arises because practitioners of these disciplines are looking for a means or a way by which they can increase their capacity to help their patients. Radionics clearly holds out the promise of being just what they are looking for, in that it provides a means of detecting causative factors in disease which would go unnoticed in standard physical and clinical examinations. Besides this obvious advantage it also offers another approach to treatment which can be utilised as an adjunct to the more physical theraputic agents normally employed, and directed specifically towards the elimination of hidden causative factors which so often lie behind chronic problem cases.

If radionics holds out such obvious advantages, why then do the majority of health care professionals who investigate this approach to healing, frequently and often quickly lose interest and look elsewhere — what is it that deters them? I have seen all too many doctors who may have benefitted from the use of radionics in their practices, or who may have been able to contribute their ideas to this healing art, lose interest. If you ask them why they are no longer giving radionics serious consideration, they invariably reply that apart from one or two personal reasons, there are certain factors that put them off. The prime one seems to be the numerous and often conflicting belief systems that operate in radionics, and the second is the element of time involved in often over complicated methods of diagnosis and treatment. Both of the problems are of course overcome if the enquiring practitioner is prepared to shoulder aside the burden of first impressions and take a look at the basic premises that underlie the theory and practice of radionics.

Before dealing with the basic premises of radionics and outlining a method of practice that can be utilised by the health care professional, I think it will be of benefit to range briefly through the development of radionics and to highlight one or two of those aspects that tend to deter the serious investigator from further enquiry.

During the formative and pioneering years of radionics at the beginning of this century, right through the 1930's and even into the late 40's, the list of practitioners who utilised radionics in one form or another read like a "Who's Who" of the healing arts. Apart from Dr. Albert Abrams, whose perceptive mind and genius gave birth to what we now call radionics, there was Dr. Thomas Colson an osteopath who contributed much to this branch of healing through his researches and teaching, and his close association with Dr. Abrams. McMannus was another leading light whose name still comes up in discussions relative to natural healing methods, and many clinics in America today use the spinal adjusting table he designed. From the legions of medical doctors, chiropractors and osteopaths who used radionics in their practices at that time, there was one who emerged head and shoulders above the rest to contribute as much, if not more than the founder. Her name was Ruth Drown, a chiropractor who practiced in Hollywood, California. It was she who was to demonstrate to the world that patients could be treated at a distance, and perhaps even more remarkable, that photographs of disorders in the etheric body could be taken over distances of many thousands of miles by means of her invention, the Radio-Vision camera.

The work of Abrams caught the imagination of many British physicians, not least among them was Sir James Barr who made a thorough study of Abram's discoveries and used them extensively in his practice. In his book *Abrams' Methods of Diagnosis and Treatment* he reflects that in Abrams he had found a man after his own heart, whose aim was not merely to improve the diagnosis and treatment of disease, but to prevent it. A number of British doctors went to San Francisco to study directly under Abrams and were greatly impressed not only by the man but with what he had to teach.

It was clear to them that his work contained the seeds of an important step forward in medicine. Of all the doctors in Britain who were interested in Abram's work, Guyon Richards must have been the most tireless researcher. His persistence in facing problems that arose during the course of his work, and seeking solutions that would enable him to help his patients more fully, is most evident when one reads his book *The Chain of Life* which contains a great deal of useful information and historical background in this field for any doctor who may be contemplating using radionics in its present form.

There were other physicians too, like Dudley Wright, Ernest Martin, Hector Monroe, Ernest Jensen, Hugh Wyllie and Winter Gonin who developed the theory and practice of herbal hormone therapy, Aubrey Westlake whose book *The Pattern of Health* is a classic in the field of medical radiesthesia, and will no doubt remain so for a long time to come. Dr. George Laurence another physician of wide experience was attracted to this field and his researches gave rise to what is known today as Psionic Medicine, an approach to healing through the use of the radiesthetic faculty and homoeopathy, which amongst other things offers hope for the very many who suffer from the adverse affects of hereditary and acquired miasms and toxins, and the frequently devastating side-effects of vaccination. Along with other notables like Dr. T. Watson and Dr. Michael Ash, these pioneers formed themselves into a very active group known as The Medical Society for the Study of Radiesthesia.

So it is evident that in the early days the bulk of practitioners using radionics and medical radiesthesia were drawn from the ranks of medicine, chiropractice and osteopathy. The lay practitioners were not too numerous and tended to remain in the background of the movement. From the very beginning Abrams met a great deal of resistance to his ideas from more orthodox practitioners, and this resistance was soon to escalate into outright opposition accompanied by unjustified attacks, not only on his work but on his character as well. Soon those authorities associated with health joined in and sustained their attack right into the early 1960's when they succeeded in jailing the then seventy year old Ruth Drown on fraud charges. She was soon to die from a heart attack, no doubt brought on by the stress she was subjected to during this time.

Radionics was then made illegal by law in America and ridiculed as outright quackery. Practitioners found agents from various bureaus entering their offices, confiscating their equipment which was then destroyed. Naturally there was an exodus and many stopped using radionics altogether; a small minority went underground in order to avoid persecution.

In Britain, Abram's work also met with considerable opposition which no doubt discouraged many doctors from fully investigating what he had to offer. The Horder report made in 1924 which purported to deal with the committee's findings on Abrams work, said: "The fundamental proposition underlying the Electronic Reaction of Abrams (E.R.A.) is established to a very high degree of probability." But nothing was done to encourage doctors to look into it for themselves, which just goes to show how a technique of diagnosis and treatment which could have revolutionised medicine was allowed to fall by the wayside.

The pressures of ridicule and persecution over the years both in America and Britain had the effect of reducing the number of health-care professionals using radionics and radiesthetic methods, but a steadily growing band of lay-practitioners had taken up the work, especially here in England. Their displacement of the medical doctors seemed to be signalled between 1946 and 1950 when the Society for the Study of Medical Radiesthesia lost Jensen, Wright, Monroe, Martin, Hort, Wyllie and Guyon Richards. In his tribute to these men, Dr. Michael Ash said that although these fathers of a new age in medicine were dead, their work would live on. The appearance of George de la Warr on the radionic scene coincided with this increase in the number of lay-practitioners, and there can be little doubt that the work carried on at the De La Warr Laboratories sustained and increased the forward momentum of radionics, thus encouraging many to enter this field of healing and render great service to countless people who were suffering from bad health.

What in effect happened is that radionics having come to birth in the field of medicine, then passed into the hands of the lay-practitioner where it has been largely sustained and nurtured ever since. I believe it is here that a number of factors that discourage doctors from seriously considering radionics have managed, to attach themselves to this healing art. It is my contention that if these impediments are pointed out and then seen to be superfluous, a greater number of doctors who come to investigate radionics will stay to incorporate it into their practices in one way or another. It is essential to look beyond the appearance of radionics to the underlying reality which is simple and straightforward, useful and effective.

Radionics today is at best a fringe medicine technique, and as such naturally appeals to those who think along natural healing lines. In so far as this goes, it is just fine, but the fringe thinkers have even more unorthodox brothers who may be called the fringe of the fringe, and it is their beliefs and ideas which when added to radionics tend to frighten off the serious student, lay and orthodox alike. Had radionics remained within the orthodoxy of medicine for example, many, if not all of the weird accretions that have attached themselves would not today exist, and a healing art born out of clinical and scientific disciplines would have been in operation.

One of the first things that can repell the orthodox doctor in the early stages of his investigations into radionics, is the often bewildering array of belief systems that operate in this field. Many of them arise out of the subjective nature of radionics and patterns of ritual which are common to both orthodox and unorthodox methods of healing. Although we may not think of it in these terms, ritual is a fundamental basic of all healing arts, be they medicine, chiropractic, osteopathy or radionics. The ritual of case history taking for example, is one in which an interplay and exchange of energies and information is set up between the doctor and his patient. This proceeds into the rituals of examination, x-ray photography and clinical tests, which are essential factors in building a common area of understanding between the parties concerned. Once this is clearly defined and established, the ritual of treatment follows, which may well take the form of surgery, drug ingestion or injection, massage, manipulation, acupuncture or whatever techniques are called for in any particular case. Whichever way you look at it, ritual is involved. In orthodox practice this ritual proceeds along physically recognised lines. For example a broken bone is gently palpated, x-rayed, set, placed in plaster and then rested. All things being equal, a healing of the break will result. The whole process is a clear sequence of objective and observable factors. This is the kind of thing a doctor is used to dealing with, and it is in stark contrast to what he encounters when he first touches upon radionics.

As I have mentioned before, radionics by its very nature deals mainly with subjective factors, and there is little if any, firm and familiar ground for the doctor who is used to objective procedures, to put his feet upon. The very act of making a diagnosis at a distance contains so many intangibles that some can't even get by this first hurdle, let alone come to terms with treatment at a distance. Those who can accept these concepts and press on with their investigations inevitably run into some of the more bizarre beliefs which many lay-practitioners entertain and subscribe to at one time or another. These often arise out of the subjective nature of radionic procedures, which can at times get out of hand to the point where shades of superstition and magic begin to enter the process and procedures of diagnosis and treatment.

It is worth pausing for a moment to consider how this comes about. The successful use of any technique in any healing art depends to a greater or lesser degree upon the belief that the practitioner has in what he is doing. Surprisingly this applies to medicine much more than many people realise and in a subjective procedure like radionics it is absolutely paramount. Belief in what he is doing, linked to enthusiasm, a good knowledge of the clinical and basic sciences, plus a fine degree of sensitivity are the essentials that a lay-practitioner needs if he or she is to be successful in practice. The Theosophical Medical Research Group in their book 'The Mystery of Healing' touch on this point:

> Hence it follows that the accuracy or inaccuracy of diagnosis by radiesthesia will depend upon all the usual factors involved in psychic and in medical work — experience, impersonality, and the conscious or unconscious psychic capacities of the operator. Favourable and unfavourable psychic conditions, including the resistance or sympathy or expectation of the patient, as well as the clarity or complexity of the case, must all be included among the modifying factors.

Of all things sensitivity is prone to fluctuate because it depends upon, and is directly linked to, factors liable to make it diminish. Poor health, fatigue, stress situations, noisy environment and weather conditions may all in one way or another reduce sensitivity. When sensitivity diminishes, results tend to follow suit, diagnosis becomes inaccurate and treatment less effective. This in turn drains away enthusiasm and a cycle may be set in motion in which the operator is rendered temporarily ineffective. What often occurs at this point is, that instead of recognising what has happened and easing off as he should in such circumstances, the practitioner casts around for some esoteric way of overcoming the energy deficiency. Intuitively, but more likely as the result of using his pendulum in a question and answer session, he comes up with the idea of placing a small phial of honey on the treatment plate of his instrument. This procedure may be convincing enough to release sufficient energy to get him going again, and soon reports from patients tend to substantiate his belief in the phial of honey, and before you can look around, practitioners all over the country are adopting the same technique just as a matter of course.

Another practitioner in a similar state of low energy may determine that the cause of his plight lies in malefic influences flowing from such diverse places as the bowels of the earth, outer space or from those antagonistic to his work (quite a number of practitioners think that their work is important enough to attract the attention of the 'dark forces'). The next thing you know is that the operator's radionic instrument is plastered with stickers bearing 'magic numbers', or that he is waving a bit of oriental bric-a-brac in the air to drive away those forces he feels are interfering with his work, or disturbing his own energy fields. One radiesthetist for whom I had the greatest respect, developed the disconcerting habit of frequently getting up in the middle of quite ordinary conversations, taking out his pendulum, swinging it a few times and then rearranging the position of a beautiful cut-glass bowl that stood on a table in the corner of the lounge. Apparently it was his belief that this object was radiating energies into the room, and was in need of re-positioning from time to time.

These are just one or two examples of the peculiar beliefs and practices that enter into radionics, there are dozens of others. I once had in my possession two radionic treatment sets that had formerly belonged to a Reverend gentleman; Yes, as you've probably guessed instead of the standard rectangular shape, they were built in the form of pulpits. Personalised pendulums are another peculiar belief which is adhered to by a number of practitioners, and some have made a great deal of money from exploiting this superstition. The fact is a pendulum works no matter what. Then there are of course those who would not go near a perspex pendulum, their claim is that it is not a natural product like wood or whale bone, therefore it is inferior and will not respond as well. I always used a perspex pendulum and I have never seen Malcolm Rae use anything else, and it has never made any difference whatsoever to us, nor to hundreds of others who do not subscribe to the belief that a natural pendulum is a better pendulum. Of course if it is essential for the practitioner to prop up his belief system, or to complicate it with personalised or natural pendulums then no real harm is done, except to the objective observer it makes no sense at all, and in some cases it will cause him to turn his back on radionics, convinced that its practitioners are a rather odd lot and that the system has little to offer.

Another unfortunate aspect of radionics that can put off the health-care professional, are the cult groups. These are formed by people who have a tendency to gather around a radionic practitioner who has developed a technique which he imbues with an aura of mystery or super-effectiveness. Being a member of such a group calls to some degree or other for a peculiar kind of obedience. What the teacher says becomes gospel, even if it contradicts factual evidence or flies directly in the face of truth and utilises flagrantly ritual magic practices. In these groups a power hierarchy inevitably arises because the leader, or chief pendulum twiddler, begins by putting certain areas of diagnosis and treatment out of bounds to his acolytes. The technique is to then gradually allow certain of his favoured disciples to enter and work in these areas, thus bestowing upon them an imaginery edge over the rest of the group. The procedures that grow out of such outmoded Piscean attitudes are as a rule, long and complicated, employing all manner of equipment, thus fortunately making it impossible for the serious investigator from the health-care professions to even remotely consider the use of such methods.

Radionics is not alone when it comes to peculiar belief systems. Spiritual healing being another subjective approach to the cure of disease also exhibits similar patterns. Lawrence Le Shan in his book 'The Medium, the Mystic, and the Physicist' relates that when he began a study of a group of "serious psychic healers" including such people as Harry Edwards, Agnes Sanford, Alga and Ambrose Worrall, Edgar Jackson, Paramahansa Yogananda, Katherine Kuhlmann and others, he found that their behaviour fell into two distinct classes. The first class Le Shan defined as "idiosyncratic behaviours," that is, behaviours exhibited by one or several of the healers. The second class he called "commonality behaviours," which were engaged in by all healers. The latter it seemed were relevant to the healing effect. In radionics one would see that instrumentation, pendulum or 'stick pad' detectors, and diagnostic and treatment procedures based on the physical and subtle anatomy would be commonality factors, whereas phials of honey, magic stickers, "you must not treat the crown chakra because my guru says so," or the instrumentation won't work unless the master puts a 'fluence on it, can all be listed as idiosyncratic and ultimately damaging to the image of radionics. If the serious investigator will take the time to sort out the peculiarities and see them for what they are, he or she will find underneath an approach to healing that is worthy of consideration.

Once this has been done the next fundamental deterrent to present itself, is the factor of time. Few, if any of the doctors or natural health practitioners I know, have the time to run a radionic practice in conjunction with the discipline they have been trained for. This brings up the question of just how can a busy doctor make use of radionics? The answer will to a very great extent depend upon just how much he wishes to use it as an adjunct in his practice. If extensive application of radionic procedures is contemplated then it becomes necessary to find an assistant who is a competent lay-practitioner, one not prone to develop "idiosyncratic behaviours," and who can be depended upon for consistent and accurate performance. On the other hand if just the odd difficult cases are going to be checked by radionic means, the doctor may have time to do it himself, or alternatively he may ask a full-time radionic practitioner engaged in his own practice, to do the checking for him. Some doctors like to deal with a small group of patients themselves, making the diagnosis and giving radionic treatments. This procedure works well, and is one I employed from time to time. Care must be taken however not to succumb to the temptation of taking on just one more patient. The load has a way of escalating rapidly and it is easy to find too much work on hand and time too short to deal with it. One aspect of radionics that can be used to the full by any doctor, to great advantage is of course remedy preparation and remedy simulation. Numerous doctors throughout the world are recognising the advantages of these radionic techniques and employing them in their practices. I shall cover this in detail in a later chapter because it is one of the most important factors of modern day radionics.

Time, or rather the lack of it, is also a problem for the full-time lay-practitioner. Originally many gradually drifted into full-time practice without pressure to earn a living from their work. Finally success as a practitioner meant in some instances that radionics took first place as a source of income. This type of slowly developing situation seemed to encourage the accumulation of unnecessarily lengthy and complicated techniques, which wasted much time and often left the practitioner very tired by the end of the day. Having evolved slowly this type of practice tends to submerge the practitioner, and block out any solutions that might help him or her to utilise time more efficiently. It is safe to say that in the bulk of radionic practices today there is a great deal of time and practitioner's energy wasted simply because they have not been inclined to question the way they work, and so determine if they are making the best use possible of their time and energy. This of course decreases their capacity to carry a sufficiently high patient load and to make a reasonable living. Admittedly many are not under pressure to earn a living from radionics, particularly where the husband is the main bread winner, or the individual has another source of income. Both of these situations allow inefficient methods to be employed without unduly distressing the practitioner and causing him or her to question practice procedures.

This kind of inefficiency in a radionic practice may not necessarily deter the health-care professional, but there is a section of those who investigate radionics who are more deeply affected by it. They are the young people who are quick to intuit that radionics has a lot to offer in that it is a healing art that will enable them to employ their depth of sensitivity and put it to good use in the service of others. This new generation brings with it a capacity to immediately comprehend the scope of radionics, and to see in it the seeds of a New Age medicine, oriented towards life and not mechanisation. I have seen them time and again thrilled by their discovery of radionics, eager to enter the field on a full-time basis, only to drift away disillusioned and discouraged by what they see and hear. In organisations where they did not expect to find it, are miles of bureaucratic radionic red tape coupled to ultra-conservative and condescending attitudes. Principles of practice that they could grasp in a few hours are tediously fed to them over a period of years, if they manage to stay the course. They run the gamut of conflicting belief systems, and it becomes clear because they are told so, that it is hard to make a living at radionics. Because of factors like these, many talented, capable and sensitive young people are lost to radionics, yet it is they who are perhaps more important than the doctor who might use such methods simply as an adjunct to his regular work. Potentially they are full-time practitioners, who with a good grounding in the basic and clinical sciences, linked to an ability to employ radionic methods of diagnosis and treatment, could work full-time as radionic assistants to doctors or chiropractors or osteopaths. This is a whole branch of radionics that is almost totally unexplored, and I am sure that a good, young radionic practitioner has a future in this field. I recall that frequently when I tried to cope with radionics as well as my chiropractic practice, I wished that there was some way that I could find an assistant to take care of those patients wanting radionic care. It is my belief that any young person blessed with a good measure of sensitivity and common sense, who is not burdened with the traditions of establishment belief systems, has a future in this field as a full-time practitioner, provided they employ a simple and effective radionic technique, and are willing to accept the great responsibility that this work entails.

In my own early work in radionics I sought to simplify technique to an absolute minimum, relying on my knowledge of the subtle bioenergic systems of man to bring this about. As a chiropractor my approach grew out of an understanding of man which was more energy-oriented than mechanistic. Chiropractic, despite what many of its proponents say, has very deep roots in ancient esoteric tradition. The profession has mistakenly, but understandably in these times, sold its esoteric heritage down the river in the hope of obtaining scientific recognition, whatever that might be. It also severed its deep ties with radionics as part of the sell-out. The trend today however is flowing back towards the recognition of values and beliefs held in the pioneering days of chiropractic which coincided with those of radionics.

The one overwhelming factor that emerged from my researches in radionics, was that there is a need for absolute simplification. This may well have been the common belief that drew Malcolm Rae and I together to exchange ideas. All his research into radionics has been motivated by the need to arrive at what he calls 'the essential simplicity', and he has always sought to simplify his methods and increase their effectiveness. He has been fortunate too in that a lot of his experimental work has been carried out in collaboration with medical doctors who are keenly interested in radionics and know its problems in relationship to medicine.

From experience we hold the belief that if radionics is going to have any appeal for the health-care professional or for the potential full-time lay-practitioner, it must conform to the following pattern.

1. Diagnostic and theraputic techniques must be simple yet comprehensive, dealing with the total man in terms of his physical and subtle aspects.
2. Radionic instrumentation must be simple and compact in design and construction, and conform with the principles of the energy fields wherein it is meant to work.
3. Proceedures of diagnosis and treatment and instrumentation must be devoid of all idiosyncratic additions.
4. The practitioner must have a solid grounding in both the material and spiritual sciences, for both are necessary to this form of healing.

If these requirements are met, then a simple and effective approach to radionics emerges which can be accepted and employed by doctors, chiropractors and osteopaths for use in their own fields, and also for use by the full-time lay-practitioner who may work as an assistant or run his own practice.

It is hoped that what follows will provide the serious investigator with a basic approach to radionic practice in terms of principles, technique and instrumentation. In addition to this, the book is designed as a reference manual for the practitioner, which he or she can turn to in the course of daily practice for information on colour therapy, remedies, the subtle bodies of man and so forth. There will be material on the subtle anatomy of man that was not dealt with in the first two books of this series, especially with regards to the shifting focus of energies from the lower to the higher chakras and their effects upon health. While more detail will be given I shall adhere throughout to the principle of 'the essential simplicity'.

CHAPTER TWO

The Field of Mind

We begin to suspect that the stuff of the world is mind-stuff.

The Nature of the Physical World
Sir Arthur Eddington

Wherever one searches through the Mystery Teachings that have been guarded down the ages by various esoteric schools throughout the world, a clearly defined theme emerges that states unequivocally that our universe is the outward expression of a vast intelligence, the product if you like, of the Universal Mind. In the Proem of her book *The Secret Doctrine*, Madame Blavatsky wrote:

> There is one Boundless Immutable Principle; one Absolute Reality which antecedes all manifested conditioned Being. It is beyond the range and reach of any human thought or experience.

Many centuries before the appearance of the Theosophical movement, the Chinese sage Lao Tsu expressed a similar concept in the Tao Te Ching:

> The nameless was the beginning of heaven and earth

Theosophy goes on to say that the manifested Universe is contained within this Absolute Reality and is seen to be a conditioned symbol of it, giving rise to three aspects or basic creative principles which it calls the Precursor of the Manifested, the Spirit of the Universe and the Universal World-Soul. From these three principles there issues forth countless Universes, Solar Systems and Manifested Stars, each Solar System being the embodiment of an Intelligent Creative Life, containing within it the pattern of the three aspects which it carries forward from the precursor of the Manifested. In Christian theology these are known as the Father, Son and Holy Spirit; other schools of thought refer to them as Positive energy, Equilibrised energy and Negative energy or quite simply and descriptively, Life, Consciousness and Form. All three are inter-related and comprise the vast ocean of cosmic energies that give rise to and sustain life as we know it.

This proliferation of principles and forms emerging from an incomprehensible source is not by any means confined to the Theosophical tradition. In Book Two of the *Tao Te Ching* we again find a similarity when Lao Tzu writes:

> The way conceals itself in being nameless. It is the way alone that excels in bestowing and in accomplishing.
> The way begets one; one begets two; two begets three; three begets the myriad creatures. The myriad creatures carry on their backs the yin and embrace in their arms the yang and the blending of the generative forces of the two.

Essentially the field of mind is the world soul and it is to be found in all esoteric tradition. Naturally different cultures and their belief systems have given rise to various models of the field, some are crude and over-simplified, others complex and heavily veiled in symbolism; a few are outright distortions of the basic theme, the product of over-imaginative aspirants to wisdom. Radionics, and indeed most subjective forms of healing are more effective if the practitioner has a knowledge of the field of energies in which he is working. In short the practitioner will be better equipped to carry out his discipline if he has a basic understanding of the field of mind, and particularly the radionic practitioner, because radionics is in the final analysis an instrumented form of mental healing. Of course many practitioners have worked successfully for years with no such background knowledge, but my feeling is that as radionics gains recognition as an aspect of parapsychology, then it will very important to have such knowledge to enable us to learn how radionics works, and how it relates to other forms of healing.

As there are a number of models of the field of mind, which particular construct is going to be accurate and suitable for the practitioner in radionics — what yardstick can be applied in order to make a good choice? I think that just as Le Shan looked for the 'commonality behaviours" essential to the healing effect in the work of the practitioners he studied, we are bound, for the sake of clarity, to apply the same process to the different models of the field of mind. We must look for the "commonality of factors" and seek where there is agreement, learning in this process to determine the "idiosyncratic factors" which have been built in by this guru or that guru, or because 'my Master says this or that'. There are authorities in the basic spiritual teachings of the world, the Bible, the Vedas, the Upanishads and the Tao to name a few which are superior to any latter day promoters of truth. If you find agreement there, you can dismiss the self-styled, so called authority who peers at reality through the distorting mirror of his own thought patterns.

From study and experience in this particular area during the past seven years or so, both from the point of view of meditative practices and healing, I have found that the model put forward by Theosophy, and presented later in much greater detail by Alice A. Bailey in her writings, carries within it many "commonality factors" and can be seen to agree with most other systems. It should be borne in mind too that this work was the latest and most up to date dispensation of the Ancient Wisdom to have emerged from the Trans-Himalayan School of Adepts. Anyone who has studied it will no doubt be aware of the Aquarian note that it sounds forth, in that it stresses the importance of reliance on the Self and not on external teachers.

The following model of the field of mind which owes much to Bailey, was presented in 1972 in a lecture by Dr. Elmer Green entitled *How to make use of the field of mind Theory.* This lecture was given under the sponsorship of The Academy of Parapsychology and Medicine at Stanford University in California. The diagram was originally developed to illustrate and ex-

plain the relationship between Freud's and Jung's ideas about
the mind, and then over the years other aspects were added in
order to expand upon the initial theme. When Elmer Green
lectured in England during the 1974 May Lectures I brought up
the question in discussion with him, of the differences that exist
between various models of the field of mind. He pointed out that

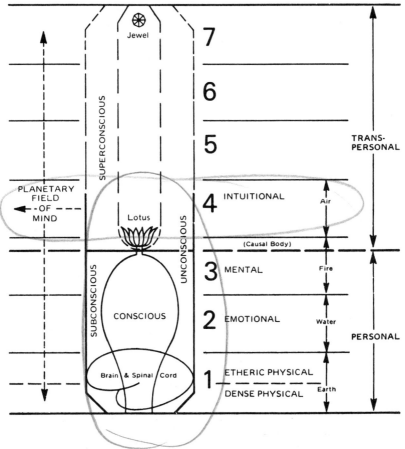

A symbolic Interpretation of Man's Substance
and Perceptual Structure.

some of these occurred because of semantic rather than actual structural differences, but it was clear to him that the model he worked with was in keeping with our present day understanding of man, and was therefore of practical value. This of course he has demonstrated in his research in the field of bio-feedback at the Menninger Foundation. Personally I believe that this construct and the one Alice Bailey presents in her book A Treatise on Cosmic Fire, are vitally important to a deeper understanding of radionics, providing an area of knowledge that will enhance the practitioner's effectiveness. Bailey's model gives a wealth of detail on the esoteric constitution of man, which as we shall see later is a reflection on the field of mind.

Rather than write at length about the details of this construct of the field of mind, I think that it is perhaps best if I draw directly from Elmer Green's lecture to the Academy. In it he said:

> The most important idea about the diagram is that every line represents both a demarcation between different kinds of substance and between different kinds of consciousness. This remarkable idea is the essence of Tibetan Buddhism when its cultural peculiarities are stripped off and also represents the basic concepts of Integral Yoga (of Aurobindo), Esoteric Christianity, Sufism, Zoroastrianism, Esoteric Judaism, Egyptian and Greek Mystery Schools, Theosophy, Anthroposophy, Polynesian metaphysics and various pre-Columbian religions in the Western Hemisphere.

From this it is evident that the diagram meets the prime and most important requirements, in that it is essential, to be found in many esoteric schools of religious thought. In other words it contains many "commonality factors" which lend credibility to the outline and removes it from the realm of the "idiosyncratic".

Elmer Green goes on to say:

> The second important idea from the diagram is that the different kinds of energies and structures, physical, emotional, mental, and transpersonal, are functional parts of a planetary field of mind. Even as magnetic, electrostatic, and gravitational fields surround the planet, so does a field of mind; and furthermore, all the fields, however differentiated, are part of the basic mind field. This means that all gradations of physical substance are gradations of the field of mind. In other words, according to this theory the entire cosmos at every

level is both matter and mind, and in some way the evolution of living being from mineral matter (not dead matter in this concept) through plant, animal, and man, is accompanied by an evolution and expansion of consciousness.

Of particular interest is the balloon-shaped section called the "conscious" at the bottom of the diagram. It is shown to have physical substance (brain and body), emotional substance, and mental substance. Surrounding the conscious is the "subconscious" substance and above the conscious is the transpersonal substance. In reality says the theory, all these substances totally interpenetrate. There is no up or down. That is merely a convenience for purpose of illustration.

In the esoteric teachings each of these levels is often referred to as a plane, and this term denotes the range or extent of some state of consciousness, or the perceptive power of a particular set of senses. It may also denote the action of a particular force, or the state of matter corresponding to any of the above. What we have in effect is a field that contains various gradations or frequencies of matter/consciousness, which from a radionic point of view can be utilised for purposes of diagnosis and treatment at a distance. This theory highlights the fact that there is no separation between practitioner and patient, nor for that matter between the precursor of the Manifested Universe and all life forms. We are One. When this becomes a realisation and no longer an intellectual concept in the mind of the practitioner, he finds himself endowed with a spontaneous capacity to heal and meet the needs of patients the moment a demand is made of him, whether it be voiced or silent.

Traditional science holds the belief that the mind somehow arises out of the chemical and electrical fluctuations of the physical cellular structure of the body. Spiritual science holds a belief diametrically opposed to this, and says that the body is in effect a product of the mind. In some of his experimental work Elmer Green worked with Swami Rama who demonstrated the effect that the mind could have over the body. Amongst other things he could bring about a 10 degree F change in temperature between two points on his hand some two inches apart, stop his heart from pumping blood or in five seconds produce a cyst as large as an egg in muscle that had been previously smooth and relaxed. Dr. Green says that:

The most potent of the various ideas that the Swami discussed is contained in his concept from Raja Yoga that, "All the body is in the mind, but not all the mind is in the body". This simple phrase has vast theoretical implications. The control of every cell of the body is possible, according to the Swami, because every cell has a representation in the unconscious. Not only that, each cell is part of the unconscious. In other words each cell exists not only symbolically in mind, but also as a section of a real energy structure called mind. When we manipulate the representation of the cell in the unconscious, we literally manipulate the cell itself because the cell is part of the mind.

The second half of the phrase, "but not all the mind is in the body", is related to the extension of the mind into nature in general and accounts for parapsychological events, psychokinesis, psychic healing, and all such "scientifically impossible" phenomena. The reason science has felt these phenomena are impossible is because scientists, at least the majority, have not been able to conceive of the mind as an energy structure which interlocks with energy structures both in the body and in "external" nature.

As Elmer Green says, the Swami's concept that "All the body is in the mind, but not all the mind is in the body" has vast theoretical implications. It is clear for example, that if an individual can manipulate and influence the function of the cells in his body through the action of his mind, there is no reason why this concept cannot be extended to include the action of radionic therapy upon cell fields at a distance, because we do after all share the same field of mind.

The diagram shows seven levels of attenuated matter or consciousness. For the purpose of radionic diagnosis and methods of treatment, the lower three are of prime importance, those above are not in any way involved in dis-ease processes. For the most part man's conscious awareness is polarised on those levels designated as personal, and it is from there that he usually functions when employing radionic means of treatment. Of course there are exceptions to this which I will cover in a later chapter, and these involve the transpersonal aspects of his nature with very remarkable results including instantaneous healings of gross pathological changes.

If we hold clearly in mind that we live and move and have our being in a field of energies called the Universal Mind, and that man utilises the substances of the various levels of consciousness to build vehicles of manifestation, and that these in their totality form an instrument which can function through the field of mind and initiate healing processes at a distance, then we are ready to consider man himself as an aspect of the field.

CHAPTER THREE

The Fields and Form of Man

*Man is in fact a fragment of the Universal Mind, or
world soul, and as a fragment is thus partaker of the
instincts and quality of that soul, as it manifests
through the human family.*
A Treatise on Cosmic Fire — Alice A. Bailey

Orthodox science has theorised for us that life and ultimately
man, may have originated when a fortuitous flash of lightning,
struck an equally fortuitous puddle, filled with an even more
fortuitous soup consisting of protein molecules and general
chemical debris. Aeons later, they tell us, man emerged, staggering
out of the prehistoric slime, virtually a cosmic 'flash in the pan'
who has since perambulated about the surface of this planet
with no other purpose than to eat, sleep, procreate and finally
drop dead. Man's genius and his power to think and reason are
seen as no more than a rather peculiar outcome of those chemical
interactions that take place within his physical organism. Fortunately spiritual science presents us with a more hopeful, purpose-
ful and creative picture of man which can be employed to help

us better understand the diagnostic and healing procedures and processes utilised in radionics.

One of the most ancient texts that deals with the origins of man is called 'The Book of Dzyan.' Blavatsky translated the Stanzas from this book and incorporated them in her monumental work entitled 'The Secret Doctrine'. Later Sri Krishna Prem and Sri Madhava Ashish wrote two books dealing with the content of the Stanzas of Dzyan called, *Man, the Measure of All Things,* and *Man, Son of Man.* In the former, the authors say that through a study of the Stanzas:

> We are engaging in an active search for our very Self, Man, the most elusive and most wonderful creature of the universe. These Stanzas are about us, our origins, our development, our conscious selves and our bodily forms. No matter how obscure the ideas that are presented, nor how strange the vocabulary that has been used, the effort to grasp their meaning can lead us to an understanding of both ourselves and of our relation to the world around us in terms of values which will give a purpose to our lives and an incentive to find within ourselves the perfection we so conspicuously lack.
>
> We ourselves, with all our petty meanness, our brutal and insane cruelties, our obscenities, our pursuit of trivial pleasures, and our misguided ambitions, bear within us the seeds of that perfection.
>
> Around us in the world an assortment of voices deny the premises for such a statement. Materialists call us epiphenomena of matter; the operational theory of truth says our thesis has no meaning; biologists have referred to us as minor crustal phenomena. Actively or by suggestion the world seems bent on denying all but material values. Man shall live by bread alone. Man shall seek nothing but merriment, when he isn't working. Man shall be dust.

I have drawn this extract from *Man, the Measure of All Things,* simply to illustrate the polarities of thought that exist regarding man and his origin and purpose. The materialist shuts himself off from the wonder of his own being, life is narrow and truth no further than the end of his nose. This is a posture that finds no place in radionics, for this science of the future is broad and deep, and by its very nature concerned with possibilities that widen man's view of himself and the cosmos. Although they may exist, I have never yet spoken to a radionic practitioner who was not first and foremost a seeker after truth, and prepared to consider within reason, all things possible. If the history of man is just a few dry bones, a fossilised skull or two dating back three or four million years and a handful of pottery shards, then we are in one hell of a mess and on a track to nowhere. Personally I prefer to consider the possibility that man is a fragment of the Universal Mind, that his origins are divine, and that he has a future that will produce a glory beyond his present comprehension.

If man is a product of the field of mind, and we are to believe that passage in Genesis which says:

> So God created man in his own image, in the image of God created he him; male and female created he them.

Then we shall have to turn to those constructs that have emerged from the teachings of the mystics and seers down the ages, and there find how man emerges from the field, and what manner of vehicles he utilises in order to experience the necessary restrictions of form. In my first two books on radionics I used simple diagrams for this purpose; here I would like to use one from *A Treatise on Cosmic Fire* by Alice Bailey which gives a maximum of information and provides the key to detailed knowledge on the esoteric constitution of man and the flow of energies through the subtle mechanisms on the different planes of consciousness.

Before covering in any detail certain aspects of the subtle anatomy of man, it may be as well to trace the path of descent of the Spiritual Man. For this purpose I am going to draw on material from a book that has long been out of print, called *The Science of The Initiates,* which describes this process in a simple yet informative way. It says: The Monad (the One: the Unity) being pure spirit "falls" into matter. At each of the planes with their seven-fold divisibles the Monad gathers "flesh" around it until it stands forth clad in the vesture of the densest matter of all — the flesh of the physical plane. The man as we perceive him with out physical senses functions in a perpendicular form, but in reality he is a seven-fold spheroidal being, costumed in a concentric series of garment composed of the various modifications of matter.

As the Monad plunged into matter it loses, in ratio, the identic oneness with its primal source. The realization of its spiritual origin passes more and more into eclipse. The man is a god in

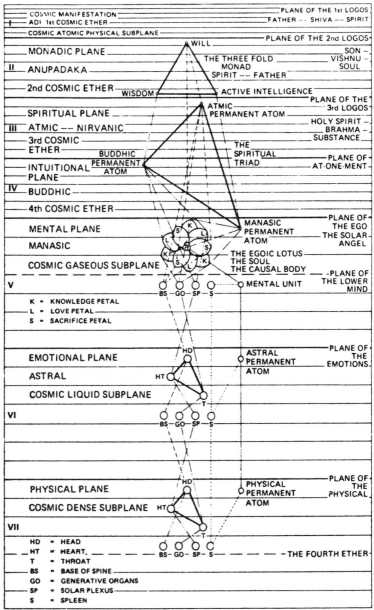

COSMIC MANIFESTATION — PLANE OF THE 1st LOGOS
ADI 1st COSMIC ETHER — FATHER -- SHIVA -- SPIRIT
COSMIC ATOMIC PHYSICAL SUBPLANE — PLANE OF THE 2nd LOGOS

WILL
MONADIC PLANE — SON –
THE THREE FOLD — VISHNU –
II ANUPADAKA — MONAD — SOUL
SPIRIT -- FATHER
2nd COSMIC ETHER
WISDOM — ACTIVE INTELLIGENCE
PLANE OF THE
ATMIC — 3rd LOGOS
SPIRITUAL PLANE — PERMANENT ATOM —
HOLY SPIRIT –
III ATMIC -- NIRVANIC — BRAHMA –
3rd COSMIC — SUBSTANCE
ETHER — THE
BUDDHIC — SPIRITUAL — PLANE OF
INTUITIONAL PERMANENT — TRIAD — AT-ONE-MENT
PLANE ATOM
IV BUDDHIC

4th COSMIC ETHER

PLANE OF
MENTAL PLANE — MANASIC — THE EGO
PERMANENT — THE SOLAR
ATOM — ANGEL
MANASIC
THE EGOIC LOTUS
COSMIC GASEOUS SUBPLANE — THE SOUL
THE CAUSAL BODY
PLANE OF
V MENTAL UNIT — THE LOWER
BS — GO — SP — S — MIND

K = KNOWLEDGE PETAL
L = LOVE PETAL
S = SACRIFICE PETAL

PLANE OF
EMOTIONAL PLANE — HD — ASTRAL — THE
PERMANENT — EMOTIONS
ASTRAL — HT — ATOM
COSMIC LIQUID SUBPLANE

VI
BS — GO — SP — S
T

PLANE OF
PHYSICAL PLANE — HD — PHYSICAL — THE
PERMANENT — PHYSICAL
COSMIC DENSE SUBPLANE — HT — ATOM

VII
BS — GO — SP — S
T

HD = HEAD
HT = HEART.
T = THROAT — BS— GO- SP- S — THE FOURTH ETHER
BS = BASE OF SPINE
GO = GENERATIVE ORGANS
SP = SOLAR PLEXUS
S = SPLEEN

Taken from *Treatise on Cosmic Fire* by Alice Bailey (Lucis Trust)

This chart represents the seven levels of the cosmic physical plane, the physical body of God. Man, as a spark of the Divine Mind has his point of origin on the monadic plane.

exile, the divine wanderer in the far country who, even in the "swine troughs", is ever haunted by the troubled and troubling dream of the Father's Home, from whence he came. In the Gnostic myths, Sophia is the divine soul living among thieves and robbers until she is redeemed by The Christ and returns to her heavenly home. The story of the Prodigal Son in the Bible gives us another similar example of this descent, followed by the ultimate return to home.

That fragment of the Universal Mind which we call man, externalises itself through the Monad; the atmic vehicle or the body of Divine Will; the buddhic vehicle expressing Divine Love, the Christ consciousness. The mental body which is seen to have a higher and lower division. The upper being the abstract mind, or the plane of the soul, sometimes referred to as the solar angel. Around this Being of Light forms the Causal body. Then there is the lower mental body or concrete mind, the highest aspect of the personality or low-self. Next the astral body and below that the etheric body and finally the dense physical form. As I have mentioned before, for purposes of radionic diagnosis and therapy we are primarily concerned with the lower mental body, the astral body, the etheric double and the physical form itself. So let us look at each of these in a little more detail.

There seems little point in going into any detail relevant to the physical body, as this can be obtained from any standard anatomical text book or atlas. However the physical form is a reflection of certain inner spiritual structures so it is worth taking a moment to point one or two of these interesting analogies. Alice Bailey writes in *A Treatise on White Magic that*:

1. Man, in his body nature, is a sum total, a unity.
2. This sum total is subdivided into many parts and organisms.
3. Yet these many subdivisions function as a unified manner and the body is a correlated whole.
4. Each of its parts differ in form and in function but all are interdependent.
5. Each part and each organism is, in its turn, composed of molecules, cells, and atoms and these are held together in the form of the organism by the life of the sum total.

Jesus spoke of the body-temple and we see reflected in the pelvic girdle with its organs of procreation, the Outer Court of the temple. Above the diaphragm lies the chest cavity or the Inner

Court, containing the heart, symbol of the buddhic of Christ principle. Also the lungs symbolising the spirit with its breath of life. Perched on top of the torso is the head or Holy of Holies, repository of the pineal and pituitary glands, organs of spiritual perception. The neck which serves to bridge the gap between the Inner Court and the Holy of Holies is an outstanding and important symbol in that it serves to point out that a 'gap in consciousness' lies between the lower and higher mental planes, a gap which must be bridged if a man is to come into conscious contact with The Christ on the buddhic plane. If we glance back at the chart that Elmer Green presented at his Stanford lectures, he illustrates it as the "tunnel" leading up into the Lotus. Of this bridge he writes:

> The connection between the conscious and the transpersonal structure called the Lotus, has many names in the East. This "tunnel," as it is often perceived in mental imagery, is sometimes called the "path," the "way," the antakarana, or Tao. In Christian and Judaic terminology it has been referred to as Jacob's Ladder. It is interesting to consider that this ladder, about which Jacob said, "this is the gate of Heaven," may represent a real structure, which when consciously constructed, brings transpersonal awareness.

Where the heart symbolised the love aspect and the lungs spirit, the throat represents the third aspect of active intelligence, these are the three prime energies of the Monad. Bailey also points out the following three correspondences.

1. Physical nature: The skin and bony structure are the analogy to the dense and etheric body of man.
2. Soul nature: The blood vessels and circulatory system are the analogy to that all pervading soul which penetrates to all parts of the solar system, as the blood goes to all parts of the body.
3. Spirit nature: The nervous system, as it energises and acts throughout the physical man is the correspondence to the energy of spirit.

For those readers who wish to follow up the various correspondences of the physical form to the inner worlds, I suggest *Man — Grand Symbol of the Mysteries* by Manly Palmer Hall, and *Occult anatomy and the Bible* by Corrine Heline; both make exhaustive and informative studies of this most important subject.

For a moment I want to return to the subject of the bridge in

consciousness, that has to be built by the aspirant to wisdom if
he is to know the Christ within. I am doing this because I want
to draw a line of demarcation beyond which radionics does not
function as such. The true initiate has over many life experiences
built this bridge that links his or her personality to the planes
above the mental level. At the point where spirit and matter
meet, lies what the Yaqui sorcerer, don Juan calls 'the crack
between the worlds', the Zulus call is the 'gate of distance', and
the Gabon natives the 'ngwel'. In the Upanishads it says of this
point:

> There, where heaven (spirit) and earth (matter), the two layers of
> the egg of the universe meet, is a space as broad as the edge of a
> razor or the wing of a fly, through which access is obtained to the
> place known as the 'back of heaven' where suffering is no more.

If you read Dr. Arthur Guirdham's books on the Cathar sect,
an esoteric Christian minority who were decimated by the
Inquisition, you will find that those who were burnt at the stake,
particularly the women, faced their execution with a total fear-
lessness which was very apparent to those who carried out these
grisly rites. They were able to do this because their spiritual
disciplines enabled them to cross the bridge or antakarana and
withdraw their consciousness from the forms of the personality,
in other words, by an act of spiritual will they vacated their
bodies which then perished in the flames while they were elsewhere. Many of these women were also healers of the highest
calibre which called for the ability to cross the bridge in full
consciousness.

This bridge linking as it does the lower-self to the higher
worlds, forms a point of power where time, space and matter
are overcome. At that point is seen the body of light we call the
soul which is surrounded by the causal body. Contact with this
aspect of our nature is of course made through the practice of
prayer and meditation, but it also happens in times of extreme
stress, particularly when a person is in the first stages of death.
A recent best selling book entitled 'Life after Life' is a study
by Dr. Raymond Moody Jr.M.D. of this phenomena in which
people have been clinically 'dead' from five to twenty minutes.
Almost all of them without exception described leaving their
body and moving or being sucked at great speed along a dark

tunnel. They get glimpses of others, friends and relatives who have died before them. Then they are confronted by what they all describe as — a being of light — which envelopes them in the most intense feelings of love and joy and peace. Through non-verbal questions this being helps them evaluate their life up until they left the body and they see in fact their whole life as on a movie screen being played back to them. At this point they have to return to physical plane life which most of them are loathe to do, so overwhelmed are they by the incredible beauty of their experience. This return seems in most cases to take the form of drifting into a state of non-awareness and then coming too in the physical body. From an esoteric point of view it is clear that these people who have 'died' and then returned, have crossed the bridge which, like Elmer Green, they describe as a tunnel. They then face the being of light which is a classical description of the soul or Christ within surrounded by the causal body.

I have covered this point at some length because there is a school of thought in radionics which says that it is possible, and in fact desirable to diagnose and treat the causal body. I am naturally in total disagreement with this concept which arises out of an inaccurate comprehension of the spiritual man and his vehicles. Let us stop for a moment and consider some of the aspects of the causal body.

There are a series of extracts from the writings of Alice Bailey in a book called *The Soul-The Quality of Life* which I would like to put in at this point in order to underline why I disagree with any system of radionics that claims it can treat the causal body.

The Causal Body is, from the standpoint of the physical plane, no body, either subjective or objective. It is, nevertheless, the centre of the egoic (soul) consciousness, and is formed of the conjunction of buddhi and manas. It is relatively permanent and lasts throughout the long cycle of incarnations, and is only dissipated after the fourth initiation (crucifixion), when the need for further rebirth on the part of a human being no longer exists.

In considering the causal body, we are dealing specifically with the vehicle of manifestation of a solar Angel who is its informing life, and who is in process of constructing it, perfecting it, and of enlarging it, and thus reflecting on a tiny scale the work of the Logos on His own plane.

> The causal body is the vehicle of the higher consciousness, the
> temple of the indwelling God, which seems of a beauty so rare and
> of a stability of so sure a nature that, when the final shattering comes
> of even that masterpiece of many lives, bitter indeed is the cup to
> drink, and unutterably bereft seems the unit of consciousness.

How any radionic practitioner could delude himself or herself
that they are treating that body which is in fact 'the temple of
the soul', is beyond my comprehension. In effect what they are
positing is that the soul or the Christ within is in need of their
ministrations, which come from the lower-self. They also appear
to assume that the Christ within can become ill and dis-eased.
This to me is completely unacceptable, and I might add that
one only connects with the soul and its vehicle the causal body
by crossing the antakarana, and when that ability is present
there is no more need to use the paraphenalia of radionic healing.

Having established where I stand on this matter, let us now
return to the personality or lower-self and enlarge somewhat on
the details concerning each of the subtle fields or bodies that
comprise this form. There are after all the ones that will concern the radionic practitioner in his efforts to restore harmony
and health.

The physical body I have touched on in a very general way
from an esoteric point of view. A basic knowledge of the various
organ systems and so forth is essential for the lay practitioner,
the health care professional will of course be well educated in
this area and familiar with its functions and mal-functions.
Suffice to say that the physical body has no life of its own
beyond that of the atoms that go into its makeup, it is an
automaton, subject to impacts of energy flowing from the mental
and astral bodies and held in one cohesive whole by the influence
of the soul as it manifests through the etheric body.

To the occultist the etheric body is the 'physical' body, and
as such underlies the dense form as an intricate web of vitalising
lines of energy. Theosophists call it the etheric double, modern
Russian scientists refer to it as the bioplasmic body, Dr. Saxton
Burr used the term Life-field which is as good a description as
any, for this body is the conveyor of forces which through the
chakras, galvanise the physical form into activity. In my other
books on radionics I may have inadvertantly placed too much

emphasis upon this body in my effort to draw people's attention away from the organic form towards the subtle anatomy, and in so doing I may have failed to make it clear that THE ETHERIC BODY IS CONDITIONED AND DOES NOT CONDITION. This statement only becomes clear when you have understood that the etheric body is the 'physical' body, and the problems that arise in it come from the astral and mental levels.

The etheric body as I have said before has one main objective, to bring energy into the physical body and vitalise it, and in so doing integrate it into the etheric body of the Earth and the solar system. At the etheric level all separation disappears, but individuality remains. Bailey says:

> The etheric body reacts normally, and by design, to all the conditions found in the subtler vehicles. It is essentially a transmitter and not an originator and . . . is a clearing house for all the forces reaching the (dense) physical body.

In his book *Letters to a Disciple* Eugene Cosgrove poses the question, What is the practical importance of the etheric body? The answer he gives runs as follows:

> It is of the importance of the true physical body to the disciple. The practical aspect lies in the centres of the etheric body and their relation to the dense physical body.
> 1. The centres lie along the etheric spinal canal. Each centre or vortex of vitality has its correspondence in the dense physical body. The important point is that the localized physical centres or organs are the effects of the vibratory action of the etheric centres. These, in turn, are the effects of corresponding centres on emotional levels.
> 2. In our physiology there are seven centres – three major and four minor. Not only have they their correspondences in the physical organism but in the planetary system and solar systemic organisms.
> 3. The three major centres are head, throat and heart. The four minor are solar plexus, sacral, spleen and base of spine.

Cosgrove makes this division of the centres into major and minor on the basis of the three aspects of energy to be found in the soul. The head centres relate to the principle of Will, the throat to Active Intelligence and the heart to Love-Wisdom. The rest are of lesser importance from the evolutionary point of view. There is no argument between this method of division and the one that states that the crown, brow, throat, heart, solar plexus, sacral and base chakras are the major ones and that there are 21 quite distinct minor chakras and numerous lesser centres of force in the human mechanism. The spleen centre drops into a category of its own as it is fundamentally concerned with the vitalisation of the lower-self, drawing in pranic fluids from the sun for this purpose, before distributing them through the other centres and the etheric body.

Alice Bailey enlarges on Cosgrove's answer regarding the practical importance of the etheric body, and I want to put this down at length for it contains a wealth of important information for the radionic therapist. Bailey writes:

> It is the centres which hold the body together and make it a coherent, energised and active whole. . . . A man can be sick and ill or well and strong, according to the state of the centres and their precipitation, the glands. It must ever be remembered that the centres are the major agency upon the physical plane through which the soul works, expresses life and quality, according to the point reached under the evolutionary process, and that the glandular system is simply an effect – inevitable and unavoidable – of the centres through which the soul is working. The glands therefore express fully the point in evolution of the man, and according to that point are responsible for defects and limitations or for assets and achieved perfections. The man's conduct and behaviour upon the physical plane is conditioned, controlled and determined by the nature of his glands, and these are conditioned, controlled and determined by the nature, the quality and the livingness of the centres; these in their turn are conditioned, controlled and determined by the soul, in increasing effectiveness as evolution proceeds. Prior to soul control, they are conditioned, qualified and controlled by the astral body, and later by the mind. The goal of the evolutionary cycle is to bring about this control, this conditioning, and this determining process by the soul; human beings are today at every imaginable stage of development within this process.

The procedures of radionic diagnosis and treatment then, are a means by which the practitioner can determine what factors lie within the mental and astral bodies and the etheric form, which serve to hamper and distort the flow of energy from the soul by way of the chakras. In so doing the way is opened for the practitioner to give very real aid to the incarnated soul by removing those blockages to energy expression which lie on the mental, astral and etheric levels. This perhaps sounds rather grand, but it should be realised that any real healing involves a change in consciousness on the part of the person treated, quite simply, he or she is able to express a little more of the Self at the centre. Ruth Drown was very aware of the importance of the glandular system, and it was standard practice in her approach to give a couple of minutes treatment to each of the major endocrine glands, before going on to deal with other problems. My feeling is that if we pay more attention to the centres of force that give rise to, and govern the glands, then as practitioners of radionics we are going to naturally increase our effectiveness.

As the subject of the etheric body automatically brings up the chakras, I am going to list here the seven major ones that lie along the etheric spinal canal, with their glandular correspondences and the areas of the body they govern.

THE SEVEN MAJOR SPINAL CHAKRAS

CHAKRA	GLAND	AREA GOVERNED
Crown	Pineal	Upper brain. Right eye.
Brow	Pituitary	Lower brain. Left eye. Ears. Nose. Sinuses. Nervous system.
Throat	Thyroid	Bronchial and vical apparatus. Lungs. Ailmentary canal.
Heart	Thymus	Heart. Blood. Vagus nerve. Circulatory system.
Solar Plexus	Pancreas	Stomach. Liver. Gall Bladder. Nervous system.
Sacral	Gonads	Reproductive system.
Base	Adrenals	Spinal column. Kidneys.

Beyond this I am not giving any further detail because it is more fully covered in "Radionics and the Subtle Anatomy of Man" and there is no point in repeating material over again when the reader can easily refer to the first book in this series. There are a couple of points however that I would like to make, the first is avoid whenever possible using the Indian or Sanskrit words for the centres and the various bodies of man. They are often long, their spelling varies from source to source and there is nothing to be gained from using them except perhaps the flexion of a few minor muscles of the lower ego. The other point, and this is the most important one, is the matter of the placing of the centres of force. One system of radionics actually illustrates their position as being right in the spinal cord, when all authentic source material says that they lie outside the body at the etheric level. Also almost everywhere you turn you come across the diagrams put out by the Theosophist C.W. Leadbeater, which shows the chakras to be along the front of the body. There are grounds to suggest that his view of the chakras was far from accurate. A contemporary of Leadbeater, Sir John Woodroffe who was an acknowledged expert in this field wrote in his treatise on the centres *The Serpent Power* the following criticism of Leadbeater's views.

We may here notice the account of a well-known "Theosophical" author regarding what he calls the "Force centres" and the "Serpent Fire", of which he writes that he has had personal experience. Though its author also refers to the Yoga-Sastra, it may perhaps exclude error if we point out that his account does not profess to be a representation of the teaching of the Indian Yogis (whose competence for their own Yoga the author somewhat disparages), but that it is put forward as the Author's own original explanation (fortified, as he conceives, by certain portions of Indian teaching) of the personal experience which (he writes) he himself had.

What Sir John Woodroffe is politely saying in true gentlemanly fashion is that Leadbeater is talking out of the back of his head, or perhaps we should say the front of his astral body. For despite the incredible contribution Leadbeater made in the presentation of the Ancient Wisdom to the Western world, he really appears to have let his own opinions over-ride the considerable body of knowledge already available on the subject. No doubt he had an experience of these aspects of his inner nature but he saw astrally rather than from the mental level, and as a result his distorted view of the centres does not accord with the facts, for he places them along the front of the body and not at the back along the spinal column. His vision of things has of course been promulgated through his writings and thus into public domain. The result is that many authors who have not taken the time to consider what he says in the light of other writings, simply use his model showing the chakras on the front of the body, and thus continue to promote and uphold this mistake with its misleading propositions. A prime example of this is Professor William Tiller's lecture given at the Stanford Symposium, entitled *Consciousness, Radiation, and the developing Sensory System* in which diagrams from Leadbeater's books are used to illustrate the chakras. Where the charts do not in any way alter what Professor Tiller has to say, they do lend credence to the idea that they are accurate, which in fact they are not.

The next vehicle to consider is the astral or emotional body. This appears as the result of the interplay of desire and of sentient response upon the self at the centre, bringing about the experience of the opposites like pleasure and pain, happiness and depression and so forth. It is as Powell, in his book *The Astral Body*, says:

> . . . being par excellence the vehicle of feelings and emotions, an understanding of its composition and of the ways in which it operates is of considerable value in understanding many aspects of man's psychology, both individual and collective, and also provides a simple explanation of the mechanism of many phenomena revealed by modern psychoanalysis.
>
> A clear understanding of the structure and nature of the astral body, of its possibilities and limitations, is essential to a comprehension of the life into which many men pass after physical death. The many kinds of "heavens", "hells" and purgatorial existences believed in by followers of innumerable religions, all fall naturally into place and become intelligible as soon as we understand the nature of the astral body and of the astral world.
>
> A study of the astral body will be of assistance also in our understanding of many of the phenomena of the seance room and of certain psychic or non-physical methods of healing disease. Those who are interested in what is termed the fourth dimension will find also a confirmation of many of the theories which have been formulated by means of geometry and mathematics, in a study of astral world phenomena, as described by those who have observed them.

Annie Besant describes this body as being somewhat similar in shape to the physical, and extending for varying distances beyond it. To the clairvoyant it appears to be a constantly swirling field of colours which surge into manifestation and then fade only to be replaced by others. It reflects the thought and emotional processes of the individual. If there is clarity and nobility of thought the colours will be electric and clear, conversely if the patterns of thought and emotional response are low grade then the astral body looks congested and filled with muddy colours. The majority of people today are polarised in the astral body, which when overactive, has a deleterious effect upon the etheric and physical bodies. It is claimed that 90% of all disease originates at the astral and etheric levels.

Mob reactions such as one sees at football matches are a prime example of just how easily negative forces can find expression through a group of people whose astral bodies have blended. The drug addict of course lives at this level, and "good trips" and "bummers" are simply examples of the higher and lower aspects of the astral plane — the "heavens" and the "hells". The vocabulary of the junkie or the acid-head provides an interesting insight into what happens through repeated use of such stimulants. For a moment let us return again to Elmer Green's chart and what he says about the various levels, in order to show how this applies.

Returning to the conscious envelope, however, it is possible to break the barrier horizontally between the conscious and the surrounding subconscious, so that one becomes aware of what is normally unconscious in him at emotional and mental levels. These levels represent the Freudian domain of the diagram since reference is not made to the transpersonal levels in Freudian psychology, as it is in the Jungian system. According to Eastern thought, especially as delineated by Aurobindo, personal safety in altered states of consciousness (which includes breaking the barrier to the subconscious) cannot exist unless one is anchored at the Lotus level, which Aurobindo calls the Overmind.

What this means is that if a proper relationship has not been established between the personal and transpersonal aspects of the individual, he or she can, through drugs, over use of yogic breathing techniques, or unsuitable meditation procedures break out through the barriers, first into the subconscious and then through and out into the extrapersonal levels of the planetary field of mind. When a drug taker says of himself that he is spaced out, there is a deep truth in this phrase, and the more drugs he takes, the more insulation will be stripped away until he finds that the whole of his personality is flooded with the contents of the planetary field. This may lead to the physical death of his organism, or at best, a place in a mental institution. All in all the astral body can be a potent source of trouble and knowledge of this aspect of man's fields is important in the practice of radionics. It must also be borne in mind that there are astral as well as etheric chakras.

The last of the bodies of man that we have to consider is the mental body. Like the physical with its dense and etheric aspects, the mental body is similarly divided into two different parts. The higher aspect or abstract mind is found upon the three top planes of the mental level. Here is to be found the solar lotus of the soul surrounded by the causal body. Bailey's diagram shows the central point of the lotus, the jewel, located on the middle of these three planes and in so doing she identifies the location of that point as it would be in the consciousness of a disciple of the Wisdom. This point in undeveloped man is on the lower of the three planes, and that of a Master of the Wisdom naturally on the top one. The threefold antakarana links the mental unit (which plays the role of permanent atom for the lower-self) with the mental permanent atom to provide a passage, or as it is some-times called the rainbow bridge (God's covenant in the sky), along which the individual may move (when he has built the bridge and gained expertise) at will from the lower levels of the concrete mind to those of the abstract mind and beyond.

The mental body is in effect that much of the mind stuff that the incarnating soul draws around the mental permanent atom, and this substance forms a body which is used for purposes of rational, logical and deductive thinking. Through it The Thinker (soul) functions with increasing effectiveness as evolution pro-ceeds. It should be noted too that only the lower three chakras of the seven major ones are shown on the mental plane, the other four are a function of the soul and are there to be found.

The school of radionic thought that claims it is possible to diagnose and treat the causal body, also states that there is no such thing as an etheric body, nor for that matter a mental

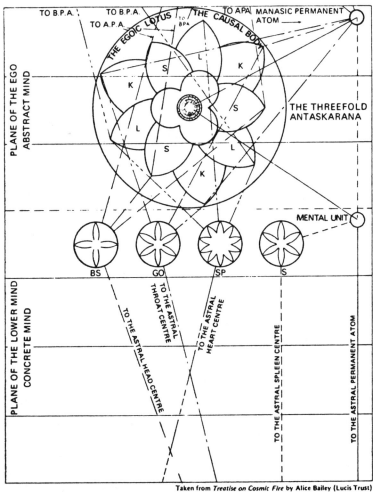

Taken from *Treatise on Cosmic Fire* by Alice Bailey (Lucis Trust)

A.P.A. = ATMIC PERMANENT ATOM
B.P.A. = BUDDHIC PERMANENT ATOM

K = KNOWLEDGE PETAL
L = LOVE PETAL
S = SACRIFICE PETAL

BS = BASE OF SPINE
GO = GENERATIVE ORGANS
SP = SOLAR PLEXUS
S = SPLEEN

THE MENTAL PLANE WITH ITS SEVEN DIVISIONS

body. Mind, they say, is a function not a body. My answer to that is, so is breathing a function, but have you ever tried it without a pair of lungs? I believe this confusion arises because the Hindus speak of man as having five sheaths (koshas) or bodies which they list in the following way.

1. Anandamayakosha.	The Bliss sheath.	Buddhi.
2. Vignanamayakosha.	The Discriminating sheath.	Higher Manas.
3. Manomayakosha.	Intellect-Desire sheath	Lower Manas & Kama.
4. Pranamayakosha.	The Vitality sheath.	Prana.
5. Annamayakosha.	The Food sheath.	Dense physical.

Yet another listing put forward by the Hindus shows how the confusion begins to enter into this matter of how many bodies of manifestation man has.

1. Anandamayakosha.	Buddhic Body.
2. Vignanamayakosha.	Causal Body.
3. Manomayakosha.	Mental and Astral Bodies.
4. Annamayakosha.	Etheric and Dense Physical Bodies.

Because the Hindu claims that man's astral and mental bodies are so closely related, he lumps them under one heading. The same process is then applied to the etheric and dense physical and before you know it you have a system which apparently eliminates the mental and etheric bodies, when in fact they do exist within this body of thought that arose from the Vedanta teachings.

Madam Blavatsky points out in *The Secret Doctrine* that these differences of opinion existing between various schools of thought, are usually the product of whatever point of view the adherents of each happen to hold. Some are simply more inclusive and closer to reality than others. Of this she writes:

> Thus while the men of Western learning had, and still have, the four, or matter to toy with, the Eastern Occultists and their disciples, the great alchemists the world over, have the whole septentate to study from. As those Alchemists have it:- "When the Three and the Four kiss each other, the Quaternay joins its middle nature with that of the Triangle," (or Triad, other), "and becomes a cube; then only does it (the cube unfolded) become the vehicle and the number of LIFE, the Father-Mother SEVEN."

In a footnote to this, Blavatsky says that certain learned Brahmins protested against the septenary divisions that appear in the Ancient Wisdom, particularly as expressed through Theosophy. She agreed that they were right to complain from their own standpoint, because the smaller number of factors that they were concerned with, were quite sufficient for purely theoretical metaphysical philosophy and for purposes of meditation. However for practical purposes of occult teaching and coming to understand the nature of LIFE (and this must be seen to include man), she claimed that the septenary division was the easiest and best to employ. I am sure that anyone who takes time to study the available material will find no trouble in agreeing with her.

It would seem only practical, especially from the point of view of radionic diagnosis and treatment, to make a distinction between the emotional and mental functions in man, particularly today when they are so apparent and clearly polarised. Few people for example, would confuse a temper tantrum which originates from the activity of the astral body, with a logically reasoned scientific thesis that is clearly a product of the mental body. I agree that the astral and mental bodies are closely knit in man, and further, that in many people today, so strong is the activity of the lower aspect of the astral body that the mental body is polluted by it. Many psychological problems have their roots in this area, where there is a bleed-through of negative astral qualities into the lower mental plane.

Likewise it would also seem practical to clearly distinguish the etheric body from the dense physical, and not lump them together under one heading, much less deny the existence of the former. No one, I am sure would look at a Kirlian or a radionic photograph and confuse what it depicts with the dense physical form. They are much more likely to think of it in terms of bioplasmic or etheric substance.

For our purposes then, and by way of a brief summary, we prefer for practical reasons the septenary division which states that man has seven vehicles of manifestation, which are as follows.

	1.	Monadic
The Three	2.	Spiritual
	3.	Intuitional
	4.	Mental
	5.	Emotional
The Four	6.	Etheric
	7.	Dense Physical

There is an ever increasing trend in psychology and parapsychology to employ this kind of septenary division in order to understand the form and functions of man and the fields he utilises and lives within. As Elmer Green points out, this model is the best we have when it comes to linking our objective and subjective knowledge of man. Those who utilise it in their approach to radionics will soon recognise the wisdom behind this belief.

CHAPTER FOUR

Action and Influence at a Distance

*The sun can shine through a glass, and fire can radiate
warmth through the walls of a stove, although the sun
does not pass through the glass and the fire does not
go through the stove; in the same way, the human
body can act at a distance while remaining at rest in
one place.*

Paracelsus

While men of science and extraordinary intellectual capacity,
not least amongst them Newton, Leibniz, Clarke and Kant have
argued the pros and cons of action at a distance, the belief in,
and demonstration of this phenomena has been a part of folk
lore and folk medicine from the dawn of pre-history. The curious
fact that a man can act upon another at a distance is a central
tenet of all so called primitive forms of healing, and shaman, be
they Eskimo, Indian or African have made use of this fact. When
I lectured in South Africa under the auspices of the Radionic
Association in 1975, Credo Mutwa, a well known Zulu Sangoma

shared the speaker's platform, and it was interesting to note his reaction to my talk on radionics and radionic photography. At the end of the lecture, he arose in full regalia and with quiet dignity said, "Do you mean to tell me that the white man is finally discovering what the black man has known for a long, long time?" I could only reply, "Yes, and all we've done is wrap a little bit of technology around it". Although prevalent in tribal societies, action at a distance is recognised in British and European traditions. Ploughmen in many English counties used to treat the object that damaged a horse's hoof rather than the injured area itself. Sir Kenelm Digby who was famous for his *Powder of Sympathy* is on record as having treated a man badly wounded in a duel, by taking a cloth soaked in his blood and placing it in a solution of the powder, whereupon the pain disappeared and the wounded man left in good cheer. Later when Sir Kenelm removed the cloth from the solution, the agonising pain of the man's wound returned and he despatched a servant to tell him he was sure the treatment had been stopped and would Sir Kenelm please resume it with all possible haste. Apparently this form of treatment was quite common, for Francis Bacon wrote it had frequently been witnessed that placing the healing balm upon the weapon that made the wound, healed the wound itself.

Today parapsychologists all over the world are taking a long hard look at this kind of phenomena. Evidence came out of Russia in the 1960's which suggested that a considerable amount of scientific experimentation was going on to determine what factors were involved in action and influence at a distance. Captain Edgar Mitchell, made public his experiments in telepathy which were carried out during his historic flight to the moon. Thus an area that was considered not so long ago to be the sole province of the witchdoctor is now under close scrutiny by members of the establishment.

The leading Russian researcher in this field was L.L. Vasiliev who died in 1966. He showed through numerous experiments that influence at a distance could be demonstrated under laboratory conditions. As far back as 1934 they were able to put subjects to sleep where they stood, simply by making and projecting mental suggestions from a distance. The implications of this are of course manifold, first it is clear that the phenomena can be used for negative purposes to influence people in ways that are not in keeping with high moral and ethical standards, and it does not take much imagination to see how this might be used in the field of politics or labour relations. On the other hand it has many positive applications, not least amongst them, healing at a distance and also to illustrate that we do indeed share a common field of experience, and what we put into that field in the way of thought and emotional energy, effects others for good or for bad.

In his book, *Experiments in Distant Influence* Vasiliev reports the following features which were very common in sleep experiments, and these indicate very clearly just how precisely mental orders can be registered by subjects at a distance. He writes:

1. The impression is created that, although mental suggestion to go to sleep and wake up are immediately perceived by the subject, the implementation of the perceived suggestion is delayed owing to an initial conscious or unconscious resentment. It should be noted that a similar resentment against the hypnotist's order is often manifested in ordinary (verbal) suggestion.
2. Questioning elicits that the percipient subjectively perceives a connection of some sort with the sender, sometimes symbolised by "a thread", sometimes "the unwinding of a reel", etc. Often mental suggestion is perceived as an order transmitted by telephone. Such details of course cannot give us an understanding of the nature of the energetic influence of the sender on the percipient, but from a psychological point of view such details deserve attention.
3. Questioning elicits that the percipient not only subjectively perceives a connection of some sort with the sender but also recognises which of the experiments is acting on her by mental suggestion.

Back in 1869 a French doctor by the name of Dusard found that he could put people to sleep by means of mental suggestion from a distance, and in 1878 another French doctor named Héricourt experimented in a similar way with one of his patients and found that he could direct her to leave the house, and walk along certain streets to a specific destination without her knowledge of what was happening.

From these incidents it is clear that the mind can exert influence at a distance. Particularly interesting from a radionic point of view is the fact that subjects in the Russian experiments knew when they were being influenced, and by whom. People under radionic treatment sometimes register the moment that they are "broadcast" to, and Dr. A.K. Bhattacharyya of India tells me that certain patients of his in Canada, know immediately their photograph is being irradiated by the radiations from gems at his clinic in Naihati, Bengal, and can identify the correct time of transmission. The symbol of a thread linking the percipient and the experimenter brings to mind the **Kahuna** theory of the aka thread which the Polynesian healers use in order to transmit influences to people at a distance. Personally I believe that we employ similar threads or energy links made up of mental, astral and etheric substance to carry radionic treatment to patients. I have dealt with this theory in my book 'Radionics — Interface with the Ether Fields' under the heading The Geometric Etheric Link, so I will not go into details here but simply refer the reader to that source.

Following in the wake of Cleve Backster and Marcel Vogel, many people have conducted successful experiments to show that plants respond to human thought at a distance. In San Jose I have watched Marcel Vogel employ a split leaf philodendron hooked to a wheatstone bridge and strip chart recorder to analyse the state of a person's chakras. Having elicited a response on several of the centres showing that they were not functioning properly, he then proceeded to give a treatment mentally to balance the function of one of these chakras. It was a remarkable experience to watch the recording pen crab sideways up the graph paper, tracing out what looked like a series of steps as the energy flowed in surges from Marcel to the person he was treating. The moment the balance of the chakra returned to normal the pen slid across the paper and took up a central position and traced a normal base line. What Marcel did with a plant and electronic equipment, the radionic practitioner does through a radionic instrument and a pendulum, unfortunately the results are not so dramatically illustrated but they nevertheless follow a similar pattern. Both methods employ question and answer in order to determine subjective factors relative to conditions of health and disease, and both project energy to bring about healing — Marcel directly, the radionic practitioner by way of instruments for that purpose.

The big question is of course, how does it work? The answer is no one really knows despite the fact that a great many people have spent countless hours theorising on the mechanics of the phenomena. In 1960, having spent many years in general practice along strictly orthodox lines followed by a long searching foray into unorthodox areas, Dr. George Laurence wrote in a pamphlet entitled *Knowing and Affecting by Extra Sensory Means* that:

> After some eighteen years of radiesthetic practice I doubt if I am any nearer to knowing how it works, or why it works at all, but I am more and more certain that the solution lies in the realm of extra-sensory perception, rather than coming within the scope of materialistic science.
>
> However, I do know, without a shadow of a doubt, that it does work, and I am convinced that it could provide the answer to countless medical problems, and could transform medicine from a somewhat uncertain art into an exact science, and so be of inestimable value in the alleviation of human, and indeed animal suffering.

Well if we don't know for sure, it is certainly permissible to theorise and come at least to some sort of a working hypothesis. In the radionic situation we have the field of consciousness containing the patient as a unit of consciousness and the practitioner as another. Normally the patient initiates the process by writing to the practitioner for help, so a contact is set up, a thread if you like now spans the apparent gap between the two, although at higher levels of consciousness no gap exists at all. The practitioner using the patient's witness can then use the thread or link to obtain information relative to the various structures, both subtle and physical. This is done by a series of questions mentally posed, and it is my theory that the question (as a thought) immediately impinges upon the field of the patient, and if the question finds its counterpart in the patient then there is a feedback of energy along the thread (which I have theorised is a two-way helix pattern) and the practitioner gets a positive reaction with his pendulum. If that factor is not present in the patient then there is no feedback and naturally no pendulum reaction. By analogy the energy charge of the question is like the beam of a sonar scan, if it strikes a mirror image of itself in the patient you get a signal back, just as sonar striking the hull of a submarine will produce a return. If there is no submarine then you get no signal back. This of course brings up the point that the signal may have just missed the target (disease condition/submarine) and although no reaction was registered, there is still a health problem present. This situation of a "miss" can occur quite easily if the practitioner does not concentrate on his or her work in a relaxed manner and maintain clarity of thought . . . woolly or distracted thinking will inevitably bring bad results. Correctly designed radionic instruments and simple procedures also help to obtain a high degree of accuracy.

There is a rather lovely commentary by Confucius on the second place of the Hexagram Inner Truth in the *I Ching*, which refers to influence at a distance and the matter of clarity.

Nine in the second place means:

A crane calling in the shade.
Its young answers it.
I have a good goblet.
I will share it with you.

Of these lines Wilhelm says that they refer to the involuntary influence of a man's inner being upon others of kindred spirit. Whenever a clear expression of sentiment or truth is made, a mysterious far-reaching influence is exerted, and the root of this influence resides in one's inner being. Confucius said of this line:

The superior man abides in his room. If his words are well spoken, he meets with assent at a distance of more than a thousand miles. How much more then from near by! If the superior man abides in his room and his words are not well spoken, he meets with contradiction at a distance of more than a thousand miles. How much more then from near by!

It requires no stretch of the imagination to put the practitioner in the place of the superior (disciplined) man, and to see the "words" as clearly and precisely executed diagnostic and treatment procedures, which will meet with assent (healing) at a distance of more than a thousand miles. And the caution is added that if the "words"/treatment are not well given then a negative result will accrue.

As I have mentioned before and will repeat again here, there is an esoteric axiom which states that ENERGY FOLLOWS THOUGHT. In *Letters to a Disciple* Eugene Cosgrove poses the question:

> What is the technical explanation of the statement "energy follows thought?"

And he gives us the answer:

> Any vibration set in motion from an above plane or level of activity is registered through the entire mechanism. The response-apparatus reacts in unison and simultaneously. When the Ego (soul), the Thinker on his own plane of manifestation, sends forth an impulse, the mind-stuff responds with a collateral vibratory action. A similar effect is produced in the emotional body. To this effect (and effects are caused in relation to a "lower body" or plane) the etheric body responds. To this response the brain reacts, vibrating in harmony with the etheric mechanism. It is the brain-response which stimulates the entire nervous system to activity. Thus the original Egoic impulse has its fulfillment in the energizing of the entire physical vehicle.

Cosgrove's answer merits considerable meditation because it reveals a wealth of information, and if the practitioner were to fully cognize the essence of what is being said, it would bring to life the concept of just how the subtle anatomy reacts to the impulse of thought. One thing that it reveals is the fact that in order to initiate any real change in a vehicle, the impulse must come from the plane or vehicle above. This means that problems of an astral nature MUST be approached from the mental plane, and if 90 to 95% of all disease processes take place at the astral and etheric levels then this will be sufficient to take care of the bulk of cases that any practitioner faces in his day to day practice. Of course this also means that disease on the level of the concrete mind can only be really effectively tackled from the soul or abstract mind level, or above. Most of what is termed mental illness today is in fact derangement of the astral mechanism, the mental body of man has not functioned sufficiently long enough nor powerfully enough to create any real disease problems for itself. This is yet to come according to the teachings of the Ancient Wisdom.

It was clear to the Russians that some form of telepathic interplay was set up in their influence at distance experiments, and this of course does happen in radionics between patient and practitioner. Alice Bailey points out that various forms of telepathy exist. On an interior individual basis as:

1. Between soul and mind.
2. Between soul, mind and brain.

Between individuals:

1. Between soul and soul.
2. Between mind and mind.
3. Between solar plexus and solar plexus, therefore purely emotional, using the astral body only.
4. Between all these three aspects simultaneously, in the case of very spiritually advanced people.

Many radionic practitioners work through the solar plexus as this is the line of least resistance for them, with just enough of the mind involved to render their work effective. Ideally the mental aspect should be dominant and the astral solar plexus aspect relatively quiescent, in this way a field is formed that readily responds to impression without in any way being involved in the flow of data. Too much astral involvement can mean too much empathy, and this for some practitioners at least, can be disastrous for their own health and well-being. A good blend of mind and solar plexus constitutes what we call the intuitive aspect in which a flow of information coming from the patient is received clearly and effortlessly. I must hasten to add here however, that from an esoteric point of view radiesthetic intuition is a blend of what the Theosophist calls kama-manas (feeling-mind or astral-mind) and the Hindus, manomayakosha. True intuition is the synthetic understanding which is the perogative of the soul, and only occurs when the soul simultaneously reaches out towards the monad and the integrated personality. The intuition in radionics is a RECOGNITION OF SIMILARITIES which springs from a clear and analytical mind as it scans through the aura of the patient at a distance.

Whatever the mechanics of action and influence at a distance may be, the fact remains that the phenomena is utilised to good effect in radionics by bringing balance and healing to the fields of man, of animals and of the Earth. It would be nice to know exactly what happens, but at least for the time being we can share the conviction of Dr. George Laurence who put the principle to good use for many years in the development and practice of Psionic medicine, and know without a shadow of a doubt that it does work.

CHAPTER FIVE

Energies, Forces and Thought-Forms

The vibration of all physical bodies of the earth, and all other parts from the earth side of Energy is essentially the same magnetically, but the animating Life Force, taken from the ether side, or the individual Life or Radiant Energy, is entirely different.
                                        Dr. Ruth Drown, D.C.

Both the orthodox and spiritual scientists agree that energies and forces make up the sum total of all there is. It is an ancient axiom that there is naught but energy and that all we see and observe around us provides evidence of this. Drown, with her extensive knowledge of the Kabbala was aware that the life of the physical body, contained within the atoms and molecules was not to be confused with the Life that pervaded and held the flesh into a cohesive whole, and this is reflected in her statement which appears above. It is really just another way of saying that the physical body is not a principle, but just an automaton energised by the forces flowing through it from the other vehicles.

Man lives submerged in the etheric body of the planet, sub-jected to the ceaseless flow of energies and forces that flood through our solar system. His chakras, each one sensitive to particular ranges of vibratory activity, act as transducers for energies flowing from planetary sources within our system and even beyond. He is subjected also to those energies which flow from the Earth itself and from the thoughts and feelings of others. His spleen is the outward expression of a direct link to the life giving forces of the Sun, which vitalise his physical form by way of the etheric double. The geometric shapes of all life-forms in all kingdoms of nature reveal the workings of the four etheric formative forces, and the book of the body of man with its seals upon the back can be readily deciphered to reveal its mysteries when one holds this key.

Thought is a most compelling shaper and director of the forces and energies of nature. Bailey says:

> It must increasingly be borne in mind that there is nothing in the created world but energy in motion, and that every thought directs some aspect of that energy. . . .

This statement is of particular importance to the radionic practitioner, who by the very nature of his approach to healing must learn to understand and work consciously with a variety of energies directed by thought. Each and every day, through the processes of thinking, we build thought-forms. Some remain nebulous and fleeting, others, if we keep energising them through recollection and concentration gather sufficient astral and etheric matter around them until they finally manifest upon the physical plane. Many esoteric sources are adamant that the entire en-vironment, right down to the houses we live in, is spun out of the mind and sustained by thought, to form in effect a collective hallucination, which is maintained and agreed to through an unconscious telepathic rapport. As this is not the place to follow this idea further, the reader is referred to the writings of Carlos Castenada and Jane Roberts in particular.

Thought-form building is of prime importance to the radionic practitioner, the very nature of his work does in fact build its own forms which permeate the immediate environment, and this occurs whether he is aware of the process or not. Obviously if the practitioner does develop an awareness of this phenomena, he or she will be able to set out with deliberate intent to build a healing thought-form of considerable power which can serve as a pool of healing force which is available at all times for the practitioner to draw upon. It also seals off the practitioner from the disturbing environmental influences which may hinder diagnostic procedures and deflect concentration on the work at hand. ✓All of us have experienced the calm and peace that pervades many cathedrals and holy sites of this country . . . the practitioner should seek to saturate his or her working area with that same kind of stillness, for from that the power to heal can be wielded effectively.

Over the years I have been able to observe this phenomena in respect to a number of practices, and two of them provide particularly dynamic examples. One is at the De La Warr Laboratories where the treatment room is lined with radionic broadcast sets, on each sits the blood spot of a patient undergoing treatment at a distance, and slotted into a clip is a card with six treatment rates and six location rates representing the areas of the body they are destined to treat. These appear simply as numbers with no indication as to what they represent in terms of organs or theraputic specifics. Every hour and a half around the clock these rates are changed by a person with no special knowledge of the rates. Now this is in complete contrast to standard individual practice where the operator knows what healing rate he is using and to which area of the body he is broadcasting it. Mentally he directs a healing energy (rate) into a given area and it is easy to understand the mechanics of this process. In the labs however there is no deliberate mental directive on the part of the person setting or turning the treatment sets, and yet the treatment is most effective. It would seem to me that at the De La Warr laboratories a very powerful healing thought-form exists, which is quite natural when one thinks of all the work that has gone on there over the years, and that the deliniation and treatment intent is set by Marjorie de la Warr, and this as it were, locks into the healing thought-form. The person changing the rates simply acts to jog the 'memory directive' of the healing intent inherent in the rates, and thus creates a pulsing outflow of healing energy to the patients under treatment throughout a twenty-four hour cycle which is repeated over and over until healing is effected.

The other outstanding example of this kind of phenomena that I have observed is in Malcolm Rae's work, where he has spent literally thousands of hours in a specific environment carrying out radionic diagnostic work, treatments and research. This has naturally resulted in a powerful thought-form upon which he can draw for treatment purposes. His quest for the 'essential simplicity' has however evolved a different approach to treatment using one treatment set of his own design which exposes the sample of each patient for a definite period to a pulsed healing influence from the 'pool', modified by the Comprehensive Ratio Card. This method is of course simpler, takes up almost no room and is naturally cheaper in terms of equipment outlay. Perhaps most important of all, it leaves the practitioner free to carry on dealing with new patients or the occasional individual emergency treatment. For the health care professional or the full time lay practitioner this is the ideal approach because any number of patients can be helped in this way without the time consuming process of constant checking and treating on an individual basis. It should be noted that the concept of 'pulsing' the treatment occurs in both of these examples and this is something that I will return to later in the chapter.

Now what factors should a practitioner become cognizant of if he or she is to build a healing thought-form that will facilitate their work in radionics? First there is an absolute necessity for clear thinking, without that the form will not be coherent and functional. Close control of the astral body is also essential, seeing that it is not tinged with negative and destructive thoughts. Cleanse it of fear, anger, resentment and greed or any other emotional responses that will clutter and render the thought-form less effective.

Determine beforehand why the form is to be built and clarify in your own mind the use it is going to be put to, for this will in large measure determine its effectiveness also. The motive must be pure and the form not used for selfish purposes.

Most practitioners that I know are involved in one way or another with the use of medication and prayer as part a of their daily life. Radionics because of its intrinsic qualities attracts this

Book.

kind of person and of course for the most part they are just the kind of people who build a healing thought-form quite unconsciously. I am sure, however, that a period set aside each morning for the purpose of sharpening the content of the form will be well repaid, for it must be remembered that a healing thought-form such as this has its origin in The Thinker or soul, and the practitioner who turns each day to the Source is replenished, sustained and guided in his or her work throughout each day.

Before closing this brief chapter I want for a moment to return to the words energy and force. There is a tendency, and I am as guilty of this as any body else, to use these two words interchangeably. In the esoteric teachings a clear distinction is made between the two, and as this has never been touched upon before in any other book on radionics, it might be just as well if it is added to the record at this point.

References to this distinction are to be found in *Esoteric Healing* by Alice Bailey who writes:

> The forces are those energies which are limited and imprisoned within a form of any kind — a body, a plane, an organ, a centre; the energies are those streams of directed energy which make impact upon these imprisoned forces (if I may so call them) from within a greater or more inclusive form, from a subtler plane, thus making contact with a grosser vibratory force. An energy is subtler and more potent than the force upon which it makes impact or establishes contact; the force is less potent but is anchored. In these last two words you have the key to the problem of the relationship of energies. Free energy, from the angle of the anchored point of contact, is in some ways less effective (within a limited sphere) than the energy already anchored there.

These few short paragraphs supply us with an interesting concept which to my knowledge no radionic practitioner has considered before. According to this definition the radionic practitioner wields energy in the true sense of the word, for purposes of healing, and that energy frequency is symbolised by the rate or ratio card he is employing for treatment purposes. This free energy is directed to make its impact upon an organ, a chakra or a diseased condition which by definition is an imprisoned energy or force. Now while free energy is more subtle and powerful than the force field of a disease for example, the latter is anchored and therefore not so readily open to influence.

This suggests to me immediately that there is great importance in pulsing the treatment energy, because by doing so, the coded instructions inherent in the ratio card or rate, do not just make a single impact upon the anchored force of the disease or organ, but give repeatedly pulsed stimulus, and sooner or later there must be some kind of response. By analogy if someone knocks once on your front door, you may or may not hear, but if they repeatedly strike the knocker then sooner or later a response will be elicited, and my feeling is the same principle applies to radionic treatments.

Another illustration of force and energy can be seen in homoeopathy. A plant contains imprisoned healing forces and it is these that are released by succussion during the process of the remedy preparation. They are released only to be transferred to the alcohol solution which will more readily give them up when ingested in a solution or on tablets. Radionic potency simulation takes free energy, converts it to force in the confines of the carrier substance, and this is released once again as free energy when taken orally by the patient.

Although this is a short chapter. I think that there is much food for thought here that can be reflected upon and put to good use in practice. The concepts of thought-form building and the distinction made between energies and forces help to round out our knowledge in a practical way.

SECTION TWO

Radionic Instrumentation

He who overturns established patterns for the sake of sensation or attention is vain, foolish and frequently destructive. He who does so because the established pattern seems inadequate, may well involve the criticisms deserved by the mere sensation seeker.

Fundamentally, a practitioner must employ the tools in which he has faith, and faith is a personal matter.

Malcolm Rae.

CHAPTER SIX

Tuning Focus for the Mind

The claim hitherto made that these machines are 'a purely physical and scientific means' of diagnosis and treatment, cannot be substantiated under the present terms of scientific knowledge. That they exemplify the working of certain laws of nature, still largely obscure or unrecognised, is certainly true.
The Mystery of Healing — Theosophical Medical Group

No one who has made a really thorough study of radionics would lay claim to the assertion that it was physical in the strictest sense of the word, nor would they claim it to be scientific in the sense that it deals with objective factors rather than subjective ones. Clearly the reverse is true, for the whole purpose of this approach to healing is to identify causative factors in disease that are hidden and do not register when standard scientific clinical tests are run.

The question inevitably arises, that if the process of radionic diagnosis is extra-sensory then why do you need an instrument?

Book.

Tom Graves in his excellent book 'Dowsing' brings up just this point, and says:

> The actual dowsing instrument is either a 'stick pad' on the 'box', or else a pendulum. The pseudo-electronic circuitry of the 'box' doesn't seem to be essential — I know one operator who just writes down the numbers on a piece of paper — but it does seem to help some operators.

I would like to add to this that I know of an operator who arranges pieces of seaweed, stones, rose petals or what have you in order to effect treatments at a distance, and reports have it that an American found, if he drew the circuit outline of the Hieronymous radionic instrument on paper and added a real prism to it, that it worked just like a constructed set. It is clear that there is a point where the operator can leave the instruments completely behind, and it is equally clear that a lot of people need them as a focal point to work through. Because they provide a step by step procedure, a disciplined ritual if you like, they act to focus the mind more strongly, which can then function within the guidelines laid down by the procedure associated with the instrument without wandering off, or without the operator feeling he may have missed something in his efforts to make an accurate diagnosis. Certainly operators who have not previously spent a lot of time utilising their extra-sensory abilities are going to find the instrument is essential.

It is interesting that during his psychic work, Edgar Cayce was questioned a number of times about the use of radionic treatments which, incidentally, he did recommend from time to time for certain patients. When asked one day, is a radionic analysis a true diagnostic method, or is it just another outfit to fool the patient? He replied:

> This depends upon the technician with same. The ability may be developed in the technician or physician using same. To one it may be a perfect attunement and get at least eighty percent of correct diagnosis, and to another it wouldn't get ten percent. It is a good instrument but (only) about one in five hundred will know how to use it.

So it would appear that there is a basis for using radionic instruments in that they provide a focus for the mind of the operator to function through, but is there more to it than that? If we go back to the quotation that heads this chapter, it says: That they (the radionic instruments) exemplify the workings of certain laws of nature, still largely obscure or unrecognised. . . . I suspect that if we return to the concept of the Universal Mind and the Mystery teachings, a clue to these workings and laws of nature will become apparent and we shall find that if there is not an orthodox scientific basis for instrumentation of this kind, there may at least be one that is respectable enough to merit some kind of consideration.

It is said that there are seven keys which open the door to knowledge of the inner realms, and ten possible keys have been listed and are as follows: Psychological – Astronomical – Physical or Physiological – Metaphysical – Anthropological – Astrological – Geometrical – Mystical – Symbolical and Numerical. Each can be interpreted exoterically, esoterically or spiritually, and these interpretations may even appear to disagree on the surface while on the inner levels there is agreement. Always the inner view is more inclusive than the purely exoteric. Where radionic instrumentation is concerned we have the factors of number, pattern and symbol which relate it to the Universal Mind. In a book published in 1975 entitled *The Intelligent Universe*, the author David Foster does a remarkable job of exploring the concept that the universe is a vast mind into which the stuff of the world is fed and processed as into a computer. He points out that in the Bible it says 'In the Beginning was the Word' and the 'Word' is simply coded information or data. He goes on to point out that all life is based on the information codes embedded in DNA, and that in effect man is a living computer card programmed with codes from some cosmic source. God it seems was an Engineer (period to 1900) a Mathematician (1900 to 1930), a Magician (1930 to 1965). Now God is a computer software-merchant, programming the hardware of the universe. Many people will of course throw up their hands in despair over statements like this, particularly the anti-perspex pendulum brigade and the 'all organics', because they see this kind of concept as one that denigrates man and reduces him to little less than a programmed cypher. The truth of the matter is that it does nothing of the sort, because the universe is in the process of revealing itself and its workings through man; technology is simply an aspect of that unfoldment. The use men makes of these revelations is perhaps another matter, but he above all living beings has been given intelligence and a relative degree of free will which if used properly will enable him to cooperate with the Universal Mind and in so doing be the key factor in what It has to reveal. People may fear computers or lay the blame for mistakes at their door, but the fact is computers only make the mistakes men feed into them, and they are after all in the final analysis, only a very poor reflection of the workings of the human brain, which as a computer is far superior to anything yet built by man. The sages of ancient China realised thousands of years ago that the Universal Mind was designed along the lines of a computer, and this is reflected in the oracle known as the *I Ching* or *Book of Change,* which incidentally is one of the fastest selling esoteric books on the market today, no doubt used by many who are disturbed by the analogies made between the universe, man and computers.

In an article entitled *Compute and Evolve* which appeared in the January-February 1969 issue of *Main Currents in Modern Thought*, José Arquelles wrote:

> To return to our original thesis, the "new mysticism" which we are witnessing is not a reaction against modern science and technology, but rather represents an inevitable outgrowth. The I Ching is becoming popular not because it is a refuge from modern life, but because its structure is once again understandable; it is now understandable because men have invented and understand computers — for the way the I Ching works when consulted, with its simple but mathematically flawless system, is much the same way a computer works. No matter what language system an electronic computer is dependent upon, its functioning is based on the binary system — the same system which, in a simplified, way governs the manipulation of the yarrow stalks or coins which are used in consulting the I Ching. It is not too extravagant to say that, in terms of the nature of the input of the programmer-querent, and of the output, the I Ching can be viewed as a psychic computer.

The seers of China clearly understood that mathematics, symbol and pattern were aspects of the Universal Mind, and that these principles could be used in order to derive information from the field of mind for purposes of dealing with life situations in ways that would ultimately enhance and expand the consciousness of the individual.

In *The Intelligent Universe* David Foster points out the following series of principles which he sees as common analogues between the field of mind and man-made electronic computers.

The first universal principle is Structure and Pattern.

There can be no doubt that the universe reveals a pattern of structure. This may be in the form of geometrical patterning, and structures in time. Structure if valid must be able to describe and communicate. Languages are a form of data structure, as are paintings or music.

The second universal principle is Data.

Data (information) is an inherent central aspect of nature.

The third universal principle is Number or Digitization.

Number is the most basic aspect of pattern or data. All human and natural data is digitized. The entire structure of nature is based upon the digitization of matter (particles) and the digitization of radiation (waves).

David Foster goes on to list three other universal principles.

The fourth universal principle is Natural Process as Data Process.

And he says that the first three principles collaborate together in the following fashion:

The most obvious attribute of the universe is that it reveals structure or pattern which is data having a digital basis. Put in creative order, the universe consists of digits or numbers that are organized in patterns of data that we see as structure.

The fifth universal principle as Cybernetic and Anti-Cybernetic Processes.

This can be related to the anabolic and catabolic processes seen in man and the universe.

The sixth universal principle as Intelligence and Will as Data Differentials

Intelligence = qualitative potential differential of data. Will = qualitative differential of actual data processing. Esoterically Will as Father links with Intelligence as Mother to bring forth the middle principle of the Son.

Although I have drastically reduced David Foster's descriptions of these principles and interpreted them in my own words with the exception of the fourth one, there is sufficient here to show that the factors of structure, pattern, data and digitization as aspects of the universal mind are of prime importance in our search for some understanding of the basis underlying radionic instrumentation.

If as the author of *The Intelligent Universe* suggests that the entire structure of nature is based upon the digitization of matter (particles) and the digitization of radiation (waves) which can be reflected in pattern, then we have a strong supportive theme which indicates that the use of radionic rates or patterns for purposes of analysing data relative to the health of man's physical and subtle bodies, is of vast importance. This is of course where the need for instrumentation comes in because the rates or patterns on the ratio card symbolise the diseases or body systems in the form of digits or patterns. The healing rate for example that Ruth Drown would have used to treat sciatica is 40.351935, which in Foster's terminology would be the digitization of radiation (waves). A part of the physical body, say the mandible 8491736, is nothing less than the digitization of matter (particles).

Radionics posits that it is possible to transfer healing data [digitization of radiation (waves)] across space in such a way that it will inform the system upon which it makes impact, what needs to be done in order to correct an imbalance. The healing data serves as a pattern or template which will remind the diseased area of its inherent normalcy or harmony. Disease then is a deviation from the harmonic of health which can be represented by a series of digits or a geometrical pattern. For example a normal sacro-iliac can be expressed by the digits or rate 849923. A diseased or subluxated sacro-iliac must undergo an alteration to its digital structuring and perhaps appear as 847913. By broadcasting the treatment rate of 849923 and pulsing that wave form we are repeatedly reminding the sacro-iliac that its digital structuring needs repair or reprogramming, particularly where the digital values have changed i.e.: the 9 into a 7 and the 2 into a 1.

The whole point of using an instrument lies in the fact that by placing a rate upon the dials or using a ratio card to represent a disease or part of the body, you have a symbol or value for the disease or part of the body which you are investigating. This saves the operator from trying to keep his mind on that factor while at the same time using it to seek out the causes of the imbalance. This point will be touched upon by Malcolm Rae further on in this chapter. People may report on those who practice 'radionics' without instruments but you seldom hear any information relative to their consistency and accuracy in diagnosis and theraputic results.

In coming to understand that geometric patterning and digitization are two vital principles common to both the Universal Mind and the theory and practice of radionics, we have arrived at a point where an explanation for their use is beginning to have some rational meaning.

The following article by Malcolm Rae entitled *Radionic Instruments and Rates* was written for the readers of *The Radionic Quarterly.* In it he has adopted the form of "question and answer" in order to convey the maximum meaning in the minimum number of words. You will see the reasons he gives for the need for instrumentation in this approach to healing compliment and enlarge upon those already given in the earlier part of this chapter.

Q.1.   What is a radionic instrument?
A.1.   This must be sub-divided into:-
Q.2.   What is an instrument?
A.2.(1) It is (to quote Webster's *Third New International Dictionary*) "A measuring device for determining the present value of a quantity under observation: (broadly) a device, (as for controlling, recording, regulating, computing) that functions on data obtained by such a measuring device".

(2) A radionic instrument is, therefore, an instrument for measuring *whatever unit* is employed in radionics, and/or for controlling on the basis of data obtained by such measurement.

Q.3.   What is the unit of measurement with which the radionic practitioner is concerned?

A.3.   It is the measurement of a thought.

Q.4.   What is a thought?

A.4.   It is a proportion, or a complex of proportions. Thinking is the activity of manipulating proportions and complexes of proportions, and a thought is a "crystallised pattern" of proportions at any moment in that process. As an illustration of the relationship between thought and proportion:- if the reader is requested to think only of the page on which this is printed, his first act will be to differentiate the page from its environment. He will, in fact, establish for himself a primary proportion of "page" to "not page". Thus, a radionic instrument is a device for measuring thought, by means of its equivalent proportions: and a means of controlling, by the application of thought, expressed as equivalent proportions, in those areas which are responsive to such control.

Q.5.   Can such a measuring instrument function without the aid of a human operator?

A.5.   No. No more than a radio receiver can convey information in the absence of ears to listen to it.

Q.6.   What sense is used to apprehend the "output" of a radionic measuring instrument?

A.6.   The radiesthetic, or dowsing sense.

Q.7.   To function, does the radiesthetic sense require an instrument?

A.7.   No.

Q.8.   What, then, is the justification of the instrument in measuring?

A.8.   For the following reasons, the combination of the sense and an instrument is likely to be an improvement on the sense used alone:-

(i)   The radiesthetic sense functions at intuitive level, and must be freed as far as possible from intrusions from intellectual thinking and from imagination.

(ii) It is responsive solely to thought.

(iii) When used with an instrument which defines the thought which has been selected for it to measure, the operator's radiesthetic sense can measure consistently more accurately and effortlessly than is possible when the operator must simultaneously create and endeavour to hold invariably in mind the particular item he has decided to measure.

(iv) Should any reader doubt this, let him test it by listening to half a dozen spoken radio programmes simultaneously, with a view to discovering how accurately and completely he can hear any one of them in the presence of interference from the others.

Q.9.   Is there any additional justification for the use of an instrument in giving radionic treatments where theraputic thoughts must be offered to the patient?

A.9. (1) Yes. To give a treatment effectively without an instrument requires that the practitioner should "hold the therapeutic thought" steadily in mind for the duration of the treatment, without permitting other thoughts to pollute it, and that he should personally provide the energy to project it.

(2) By the use of an instrument, the thought may be stabilised for any length of time, may be exactly duplicated at a later date, if so desired, and is energised without calling for any contribution from the operator.

(3) Thus, by means of "controlled devices" — or radionic projectors, — the exact nature, intensity, and duration of the "therapeutic thought" offered the patient may be reliably determined: and by the use of several such instruments treatments for many patients may proceed concurrently.

Q.10.   What is the source of the energy which creates thought?

A.10.   It is a facet of magnetism.

Q.11.   What are its characteristics?

A.11.(1) It occupies a field around every magnet, including the earth, and has an "intake" at the theoretical centre of the magnet, and a potential output around the entire periphery of the magnet.

(2) The field is believed to be an ultra high frequency spectrum of standing waves — ie. pulsations without actual outward travel away from source, containing the characteristics of every thought possible to any human, past, present, or future.

(3) It is thus possible for a brain, or for a radionic instrument programmed by a brain, to select any definable thought from this source by "tuning to its proportions".

Q.12.   How is a radionic instrument "tuned to the proportions of a thought"?

A.12.   In order to answer this, the main characteristics of "proportion" should first be considered. These are:-

(i)   Any set of proportions is unaffected by the magnitude of their components. There is, for example, no difference between the relationship of one penny to two pennies, and that of £10,000 to £20,000.

(ii) The relationship, proportion, or ratio, is in each case "one to two".

(iii) Proportion can be expressed in either of two ways, which are:-
(a)   Numerically
or   (b)   Geometrically — or spatially.

(iv) Numerical expression requires a living brain to decipher it, whereas geometrical expression can be deciphered by the application of an appropriate non-living energy. The following analogy will serve to illustrate the functions of each of the two forms of expression:-
(a)   A composer "thinks" a symphony.

(b) He writes down his thoughts in the form of a score, whereon symbols represent the frequencies and durations of the notes to be played.

(c) The members of an orchestra, using their brains and manual dexterity to interpret these symbols, play the symphony.

(d) A gramophone record is made of the performance, thus contracting it into a single unit of time, but extending it spatially along the record's groove, which contains physical undulations which are, in effect, geometrical patterns, representing the performance — representing the score — representing the composer's thoughts.

(e) To reproduce, as nearly as possible from the record, the composer's original thoughts, it is necessary only to apply to the record the requisite form of energy — ie. rotation in contact with a stylus which will respond to the undulations in the groove.

In this illustration, attention is drawn to the need for the living brain to decipher the "numerical ratios" of the score, whereas the mechanism of the record player is all that is required to decipher the geometrical representation of the groove in the record.

Q.13.   Do radionic instruments, many of which have dials on which numbers are selected to tune the instrument to the requisite thought, use numerical representation?

A.13.   No. In all such designs, as far as I am aware, the purpose of the numbered scale is to enable a pattern of known spatial proportions to be built up within the instrument.

For example "5 - 9 - 6" is set on three consecutive dials of an instrument, whilst each of the other dials remains set at 0, and the geometrical pattern created within the instrument is:-

$\frac{5\text{ths}}{10}$ OF MAX.
SETTING

$\frac{9\text{ths}}{10}$ OF MAX.
SETTING

$\frac{6\text{ths}}{10}$ OF MAX.
SETTING

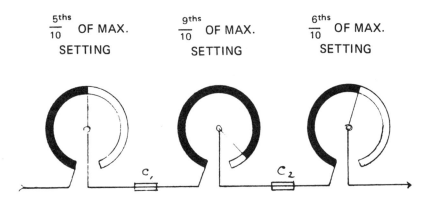

(The capacitors, $C_1 - C_2$ – or some other method, between the adjustable scales, which are frequently radio potentiometers, serve to prevent the lengths of the connecting wires becoming part of the proportion).

Q.14. Do other types of radionic instrument also use geometrical representation of proportion to tune to thought?

A.14. Yes. The two best known instruments not using dial settings are the late Mr. Butcher's "Peggoty", which uses a simple but direct method of setting up proportions by locating pegs in appropriately placed sockets, and my own design of card-operated instruments which employ geometrical drawings, consisting of a number of division marks pointing from the circumference of a circle towards its centre. A card for this type of instrument is, in fact, very much like the settings of a number of consecutive dials of a dial set instrument, superimposed about a common centre, though there are a number of reasons why the locations of the divisions on the card do not exactly match those which could be set on the dials.

Q.15. What is a practitioner measuring when making an analysis with an instrument?

A.15. He is measuring the amount of divergence between a thought representing perfection of a selected facet

Q.16.
A.16.

of his patient, and the thought pattern representing that facet's current condition in the patient.

How is this done?

If the instrument under consideration is designed for the practitioner to find only a state of balance, its dials are set to the numbers, (or "rate") for perfection of the facet under investigation, which the practitioners compares with information, carried by the patient's hair sample, of the current state of that facet of the patient. The instrument is progressively adjusted from perfect, by the slow rotation of a detuner, or "balance" dial, until the practitioner becomes aware of a point of balance between the instrument and the patient. At that point, the reading on the balance dial, indicating the amount of adjustment which has been made away from "perfection", is equivalent to the intensity of disorder.

Q.17.

How does the practitioner become aware of the "point of balance"?

A.17.

Usually by means of:-

(a) A "stick pad" which enables the practitioner to become aware of otherwise unrecognisable changes in the behaviour of the sweat glands in his fingers.

(b) A pendulum which amplifies tiny neuro muscular vibrations in his arm.

Both methods operate because man possesses responses to a "state of coincidence" between items on which he is focussing attention, and both "stick pad" and "pendulum" serve to so amplify such responses that the practitioner becomes aware of them.

Q.18.   Has either method an advantage?

A.18.   Yes. The pendulum.

Q.19.   Why?

A.19.(1) Because it is less liable to be influenced by changes in the practitioner's skin moisture, by fatigue, or by the humidity in which the practitioner is working.

(2) Because when thoroughly mastered, the combination of a pendulum and charts can make directly available

to the practitioner a much more extensive range of information than can the stick pad.

Q.20.   How is the data, numerical or geometrical, to represent a thought obtained?

A.20.   It is obtained by a trained radiesthetist who is able to set the dials of an instrument to the point of balance with a thought which he can hold steadily for long enough to perform this act: or by achieving a similar transform from thought to numerical representation using a numbered chart and a pendulum. Either method is referred to as "rate-finding".

Q.21.   Are there special requirements for rate finding?

A.21.   Yes, it is essential that the "finder" should understand the difference between "discovering" and "inventing". "Discovering" or "becoming aware of what already is" is a function of the intuition, whereas "inventing" is a function of the imagination.

Q.22.   Why is this difference so important?

A.22.   Numerical proportions and geometrical patterns may both be regarded as "symbols" for thoughts. Symbols may be divided into two distinct classes, which are:-

(1)   Those which represent the thoughts whereby the Creator of this Universe defined it, and every function and structure of it and within it. Related to any man's life, these are permanent, having probably the duration of the life to the Universe itself. They are consistently relevant, and might be regarded as the "programming" of the Universe; They are in accord with Universal Law, and can be discovered — but not invented, for they already exist.

and

(2)   Those which are invented by man. These are probably much less permanent, and will usually lose their meaning as soon as their inventor, or those who believe in him, cease to keep them alive. They are usually more complex than the symbols of the Universe.

In order to be universally valid and permanent in meaning, it is, of course, essential that numerical or

geometrical representations should be symbols of the
Universal order.

Q.23.   In the light of the foregoing, how can the purpose of
an instrument be summarised?

A.23.   Thus:-

(1) A radionic instrument is a piece of apparatus
designed to assist a radiesthetically sensitive
practitioner to do his work:-

(a)   as efficiently as possible

(b)   as effectively as possible

and (c)   as effortlessly as possible.

(2) It is not essential to every such practitioner, but
it seems likely that most of those who do not
use one would gain in overall results were they
to do so.

(3) There may be a very very few practitioners who
can function at maximum efficiency without
the help of any instrumentation, but they are
probably "artists" who cannot teach their knowledge to others, and are limited in their contribution to humanity by the amount they can achieve
personally.

(4) The use of an instrument and a standardised (but
not too rigidly standardised) method of employing it produces a basis for both comparison
of results, accumulation of a workable volume
of knowledge, and for teaching.

I think by now that the reader will begin to see that there is
a real need and justification for radionic instruments. The
question arises what choice of instrument should be made out
of the number that are presently available on the market. For
the newcomer to this field it is certainly best to check every
model out carefully, if the opportunity arises to open different
sets and to look at the circuitry and general layout, then do so.
Some are beautifully and carefully made, others look as though
the builder had found a cheap job-lot of ill assorted parts and
then hurriedly and incorrectly wired them together. Spend time
talking to different practitioners as to their particular preferences

until you feel that you have all the facts and can make up your own mind. It is a mistake to run out in a burst of intiial enthusiasm and purchase the first set to hand. Always remember that this is an area where personal opinion and choice are of prime importance, each individual practitioner feels that the set he works with is the best for his needs. You must be sure to choose on the basis of your own conviction, your beliefs and your needs, and in so doing provide a firm point from which you can effectively work in the future.

Both Malcolm Rae and I have over the years thoroughly checked out and used many different types of radionic equipment. He has designed sets with the number of tuning dials as high as one hundred, and then moved on to the elegant Base 44 instrument and later to portable variations of this design which many practitioners use today. I began with seven dials on my Mark I Centre Therapy instrument, then up to twenty one and finally back to fourteen in the Mark III. At all times we were both seeking to arrive at a design which was both simple and effective. Today the instrument that seems to fit this bill is the Rae MAGNETO-GEOMETRIC RADIONIC ANALYSER which I had the privilege to see evolving through the various stages of its development. At the time I spent a few hours of each Wednesday with Malcolm, discussing radionics and gathering material for the book I was writing, to be called *Radionics — Interface with the Ether Fields*. The book went to print before the final model emerged so I was not able to include any material on this development, which after more than two years of use by health care professionals all over the world, is beginning to revolutionise the practice of radionics. In effect this book is a continuation of 'Interface' bringing my reportage on this field right up to date, so let us look at the various facets of the most up to date radionic equipment available, covering its purposes, principles and modes of operation.

THE RAE MAGNETO-GEOMETRIC RADIONIC ANALYSER

PURPOSE:-
This instrument, intended to be a marked improvement upon its predecessors, has been designed to:-

1. Be as simple as possible both in construction and in use.
2. Be as light and compact as possible.
3. Be independent of power supplies or batteries.
4. Be as free as possible from liability to damage or to any form of maladjustment.
5. Enable any competent operator to measure, accurately, disturbances throughout, or at any specific point in any patient, throughout the entire area wherein disturbance could be radiesthetically detectable.
6. Yield measurements of reduction in "reserves of health" rather than merely measurements related to the patient's immediate condition at the moment of measurement.
7. Yield measurements, by selection, of either:-
   (a) the mean or average deviations from health throughout a system or organ.
   (b) the deviation from health at the worst point in a system or organ.
8. Yield the information required by the user, rapidly, concisely and without unnecessary measurement.

PRINCIPLE:-

The instrument employs the now well-tried principle of magneto-geometry — that is, the data is fed into it in the form of cards, representing organs, named diseases, and remedies, and measurements of the patient's condition and remedial requirements are made against these.

The instrument thus defines the information which the operator seeks, and he obtains this by the use of a pendulum over a chart which is connected to the instrument's output.

This is in effect a refinement of the customary use by radiesthetists, of a 100 cm rule along which to measure the "balance point" between a remedy and a patient's requirement for that remedy: but it is arranged to provide the basis of a rapid and searching diagnostic system.

CONSTRUCTION:-

The analyser consists of two components, namely:-
(a) a wooden box 238mm x 152mm x 90mm, fitted with a perspex panel through which are cut three slots to accept

data cards, and carrying four switches and a pointer dial.
(b) a flat chart holder, incorporating magnetised rubber sheet,
which plugs into the wooden box.
Two laminated washable charts are supplied with the instrument,
one for analysis and the other for remedy selection — but an

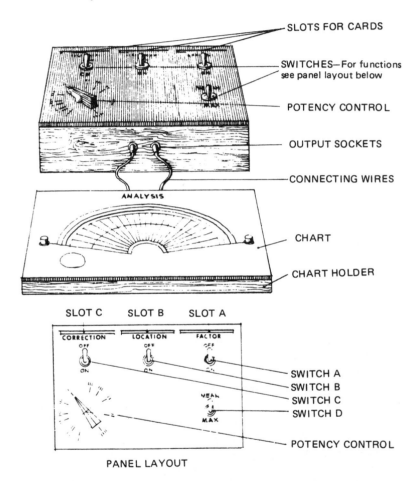

IT MUST BE EMPHASISED THAT THE OPERATION
OF THIS INSTRUMENT IS DEPENDENT UPON THE
SENSITIVITY OF THE USER

experienced practitioner may design his own charts to include specific information which he may require.

A datum card is provided with the instrument for each item appearing on the analysis chart, together with a card labelled "Symptoms of disorder". Cards for more detailed analysis, and for remedies may be purchased separately.

OPERATION:-

The analyser is extremely flexible in application, and users will undoubtedly develop their individual methods of employing it. Nevertheless, the following is offered as one effective method:

PREPARATION TO ANALYSE:-

1. Connect the chart holder to the instrument case by inserting its two plugs in the sockets provided, without crossing the wires.
2. Set potency selector at "0".
3. Set switches "A", "B" and "C" at "OFF", and switch "D" at "MAX".
4. Place analysis chart on (in) chart holder.
5. Place patient's witness (preferably a hair sealed between two circular "tacky" labels) in the circle labelled "patient's witness" on the chart.

ANALYSIS:-

1. Select the datum card labelled "Symptoms of Disorder", and insert it, name facing you, in slot "A" (Factor).
2. Set switch "A" at "ON".
3. Using scale 6 on the analyser chart, and your pendulum centred over "X", measure with the pendulum, the percentage intensity of the condition. (This may be a very high reading, because with switch "D" at "MAX" the measurement refers to the worst point of the condition throughout the patient). If the mean or average measurement is required, then switch "D" may be temporarily set at "MEAN" while a new measurement is made.
4. With your pendulum centred over the witness, discover which scale on the chart contains the next item of information you require.

5. Centre the pendulum over "X" and allow it to indicate against the scale found, the sector containing the required information.
6. This information may be either a factor or a location. In either case, select the card representing it, and insert it in the appropriate slot — slot "A" for Factor (in which event the symptom card must first be removed from the slot) — or slot "B" for Location.
7. Set the switch related to the slot in which the card is inserted at "ON", and ensure that all other switches of "A", "B" and "C" are at "OFF".
8. With your pendulum centred over "X", measure the intensity of this datum on scale 6, and note it.
9. Repeat the sequence of operation. It is likely that a "Factor" will be followed by a "Location". (e.g., "Infection" . . . "Respiratory System") — and on such occasions the intensity of either component of the disorder, and of the disorder itself may be measured against scale 6, by inserting the datum card for "Infection" in slot "A" (Factor) and the datum card for "Respiratory system" in slot "B" (Location) and setting the switches as follows:-

For measurement of Infection —	Switch "A"	ON
	Switch "B"	OFF
For measurement of Respiratory system	Switch "A"	OFF
	Switch "B"	ON
For measurement of Infection in Respiratory system	Switch "A"	ON
	Switch "B"	ON

10. Continue to repeat this series of operations until the pendulum, centred over the patient's witness, indicates "No detectable prior factor". At this point the combination of Factor and Location (e.g., "Congestion in the Physical-Ehteric body) is the primary disorder, for which a remedy should be sought.

REMEDY SELECTION:-
With the cards for the last Factor and Location to have been

found, in slots "A" and "B", and switches "A" and "B" at "ON":-

1. Remove the analysis chart from the chart holder, and replace it with the treatment chart.
2. Place the patient's witness in the circle marked "Patient's witness".
3. Allow your pendulum, centred over the patient's witness, to indicate against scale 6, the class of remedy required.
4. Within the indicated class, find the exact remedy by reference to Materia Medica, Manufacturer's lists etc., (e.g. if the class of remedy is shown to be "Homoeopathic" use scale 5 to find the initial letter of its name, and then select radiesthetically from the appropriate alphabetic section of the Homoeopathic remedy list). The correct potency may be found with the pendulum reference to scale 4.

   For those possessing a repertoire of simulator cards the following check may be made for accuracy of remedy and potency:-
5. Insert the card representing the selected remedy in slot "C" ("Correction") and turn the potency selector to 10MM.
6. Re-measure the intensity of the primary disorder against scale 7, and when the pendulum has "settled", set switch "C" to "ON".
7. The correct remedy (exact similimum) will result in the pendulum swinging to "O" unless there is a nutritional deficiency which cannot be remedied except by administration of substance.
8. Assuming the pendulum has settled over "O", the potency control should be slowly turned anticlockwise until the pendulum starts to move away from "O". The correct potency will then be indicated by the settings to which the potency control has been reduced.

EXAMPLE:-
   To augment the foregoing instructions, the following example is offered:-
Step 1.   Intensity of "Symptoms of Disorder" is measured and noted.

Step 2.   The immediately prior factor is found from scale 2 to be "Infection".

Step 3.   The intensity of Infection is measured and noted.

Step 4.   The next indication is found from scale 3 to be "Gastro-intestinal" – the location of the infection.

Step 5.   The intensity of Gastro-intestinal disorder is measured and noted.

Step 6.   The intensity of "Infection in the gastro-intestinal system" is measured and noted.

Step 7.   The next indication is found, from scale 5 to be "Mental Body".

Step 8.   The intensity of disorder of "Mental Body" is measured and noted.

Step 9.   The next indication is found from scale 2 to be "Congestion".

Step 10.   The intensity of "Congestion" is measured and noted.

Step 11.   The intensity of "Congestion in the Mental Body" is measured and noted.

Step 12.   The next indication is "No detectable prior factor".

Step 13.   The analysis chart is replaced by the treatment chart.

Step 14.   The required remedy is found, from scale 6, to be Homoeopathic.

Step 15.   It is found from scale 5 to bear a name starting with the letter "L".

Step 16.   It is found from a remedy list to be "Lachesis Muta".

Step 17.   The treatment chart is replaced by the analysis chart.

Step 18.   The card for Lachesis Muta is inserted in slot "C" ("Correction"), and the potency control is turned to 10MM.

Step 19.   With the pendulum stabilised indicating the intensity of "Congestion of the Mental Body" switch "C" is turned "ON".

Step 20.   The pendulum swings to "O", thus indicating the corectness of the remedy.

Step 21.   The potency control is now turned slowly anticlock-wise until the pendulum starts to move away from "O", at which time the potency control pointer indicates just below "M". This is the correct potency.

The foregoing may appear complicated, but the record of the example analysis is simply this:-

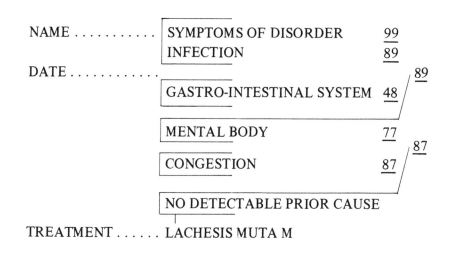

NAME . . . .
SYMPTOMS OF DISORDER   99
INFECTION   89

DATE   89

GASTRO-INTESTINAL SYSTEM   48

MENTAL BODY   77
                                                             87
CONGESTION   87

NO DETECTABLE PRIOR CAUSE

TREATMENT . . . . . . LACHESIS MUTA M

(measurements are underlined to indicate that they represent "worst points").

As an alternative any operator possessing a larger collection of cards may start from a named symptom for which he has a card — e.g. "Headache", "Measles", "Depression", etc.,
It is, of course, easy to make an analysis of all (or any required selection) of the datum points on the chart, by inserting the cards in turn and measuring each: and it is probably useful for the practitioner to check the effects of the remedy found by the "one symptom method" on other data than those used to reach it, until such time as he feels confident that the one symptom system works.

This instrument is, of course, purely an analyser, and treatments identified by its use should be administered in the practitioner's accustomed manner. Additional scales are provided on the treatment chart, to assist in assessing numbers and frequencies of doses.

The following table shows the analyser settings relative to each of the foregoing steps:-

EXAMPLE

STEPS	CARD FOR	IN SLOT	SWITCHES ON / OFF	POTENCY CONTROL AT	CHART IN USE	SCALE IN USE	MEASUREMENT OBTAINED
1 & 2	Symptoms of Disorder	A	AD BC	0	Analysis	6	99
3 & 4	Infection	A	AD BC	0	Analysis	6	89
5	Gastro Intestinal) System)	B	BD AC	0	Analysis	6	48
6 & 7	(Infection in (Gastro Intestinal (System	A) B)	ABD C	0	Analysis	6	89
8 & 9	Mental Body	B	BD AC	0	Analysis	6	77
10	Congestion	A	AD BC	0	Analysis	6	87
11 - 13 inc.	(Congestion in (Mental Body	A) B)	ABD C	0	Analysis	6	87
14 - 16 inc.	(Congestion in (Mental Body	A) B)	ABD C	0	Treatment	6 5	Homoeopathic L
17	(Congestion in (Mental Body (Lachesis Muta	A) B) C)	ABD C	10MM	Analysis	6	87
18 & 19	(Congestion in (Mental Body (Lachesis Muta	A) B) C)	ABCD None	10MM	Analysis	6	0
20	(Congestion in (Mental Body (Lachesis Muta	A) B) C)	ABCD None	M	Analysis	6	Moving From "0"

Analysis and treatment selection charts used in the Magneto-Geometric Radionic Analyser.

ANALYSIS

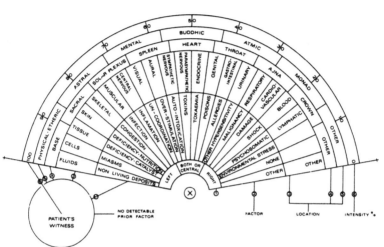

TREATMENT

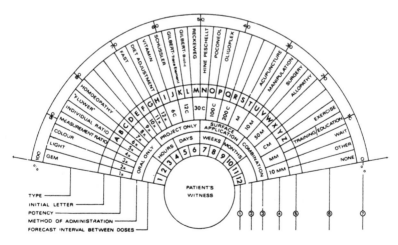

The outline of analysis given in this chapter is just one approach, but it provides a basis upon which the individual practitioner can develop his or her own ideas. The charts too can be used alternately with others of the practitioner's own design. Malcolm Rae draws an interesting analogy to illustrate the relationship between cause of disease and symptoms, which takes the form of a river delta

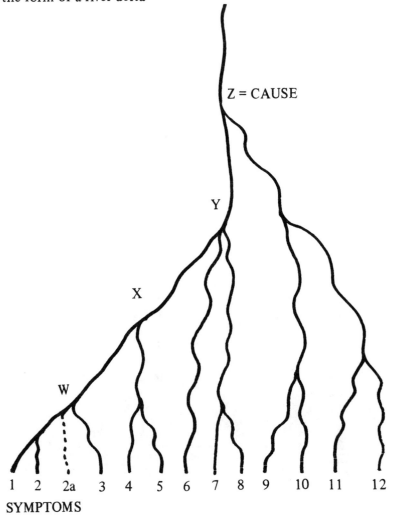

Z = CAUSE

Y

X

W

1 2 2a 3 4 5 6 7 8 9 10 11 12

SYMPTOMS

The outlets to the sea (1 — 12) can be regarded as symptoms, each of which may be seen as a manifestation of the organism's endeavours to compensate for a disorder further up river.

Treatment of a symptom alone will generally result in a worsening of other symptoms or the production of new ones. Thus is number 3 symptom on the above sketch is prevented from performing its part in the overall compensating pattern of the organism, the probability is that numbers 1 and/or 2 will worsen, or a new symptom (2A) will arise.

The approach through Magneto-Geometric technique is to take any symptom, it doesn't matter which one, and trace the underlying causal pattern. For example, the most immediate cause of symptom number 2 is "W", and the most immediate cause of "W" is "X", and of "X" the most immediate cause is "Y" and so on, until "Z" which is the cause underlying the whole pattern of disorder is revealed. "Z" is the primary point for treatment, and the remedy which is an exact correction for it is the perfect similimum, and will have a remedial effect upon *all* the symptoms. It should be remembered that any symptom can be used as the lead-in to a case, for wherever one starts this type of analysis, it will lead to point "Z", the earliest detectable cause, beyond that lies no detectable prior cause, and the end of the analysis.

This then completes our look at some of the laws of nature, particularly those of the digitization of matter and of radiation which suggest that instrumentation is of value, not only because it is a focal point for the mind to work through, but because in fact the above aspects of the Universal Mind are so clearly linked to the very process and nature of radionic diagnosis and treatment. We believe that there is a solid case for the use of instruments, and that they are not mere decorations to impress the uninitiated.

CHAPTER SEVEN

The Homoeopathic Connection

With scarcely equal opposing power, I repeat, the vital
force advances against the hostile disease, and yet no
enemy can be overcome except by a superior power.
The homoeopathic medicine alone can supply the
diseased vital principle with this superior power.
Organon of Medicine — Samuel Hanhemann

Ever since Ruth Drown devised a method for making homoeopathic remedies by subjecting sac lac tablets to various rates
on her Homo-Vibra-Ray radionic instrument, pioneers and practitioners in this field have been exploring the possibilities that
such a novel concept opens up. The whole idea that remedies
can be stimulated by means of certain radionic procedures
catches and holds the imagination because of the manifold
possibilities inherent in it, not least of these is that the practitioner has at his finger tips any remedy he needs and can make it
in any potency and amount called for. There are also a number
of other distinct advantages to this method of preparation as
we shall see later on in the chapter.

Having done a great deal of exploratory and experimental
work in radionics, it was only natural that Malcolm Rae would
turn to the field of remedy simulation. His close association with
medical doctors who practices homoeopathy no doubt added

impetus to this move, and their cooperation in the early experiments certainly helped to round out and confirm many of his findings. One thing is certain, and that is, that no one has to date devised a better method of making remedies, nor more thoroughly explored the potentials and possibilities in this area of radionics.

In terms of sequential appearance the ratio cards and the Magneto-Geometric Potency Simulator came before the Analyser that was described in the previous chapter. Over a period of a few weeks I watched the latter emerge from a grouping of three simulators to begin a more simplified approach to radionic diagnosis and treatment. It could be said that the simulator came to birth, not so much for radionic purposes but to provide homoeopaths with an alternative method of preparing remedies. In a way the simulator is not a radionic instrument in that it does not require the radiesthetic sense to work it, or make it work; all that is necessary is that the practitioner determines the remedy and potency he wants and uses the appropriate ratio card and setting. Many doctors who do not use radionics at all do however employ the Magneto-Geometric Potency Simulator in their practices, as do chiropractors, naturopaths and osteopaths. In fact apart from radionic practitioners, more medical doctors use the simulator than any other branch of the health care professions, this in itself is surely indicative that both in principle and practice magneto-geometric simulation is a proven method of making remedies that do the work that they were intended for. The fact that the demand for remedy cards runs into several thousands each month serves to confirm the efficacy of this method, certainly no doctor is going to increase his range of cards unless he has seen positive results.

Naturally enough, practitioners who use the Simulator often then become interested in the Analyser and begin to employ it in conjunction with the former in their practices. Thus some who might have originally shied away from radionics in the first instance, then find that it is a natural progression to use the Analyser to accurately determine the best remedies and correct potencies for each case that they are dealing with — the two instruments using the same range of cards, compliment each other.

Once practitioners have grasped and accepted the possibilities of the Simulator they are almost always curious as to how the cards originated and evolved, and they inevitably want to know how the instrument works. In the following article entitled *Homoeopathy up to Date** Malcolm Rae endeavours to answer these questions.

"When Dr. Hahnemann first formulated the concept of Homoeopathy, he gave to the world an extremely effective system of therapy, which has survived the test of time incredibly well — for time has been very unkind to it.

"Since the system was first developed, the number of stresses to which man has subjected himself has multiplied many times. The concept is none the less valid in spite of the extra complications in which it has become involved — but every new threat to human health requires its similimum — and it does require of the practitioner much greater skill in the selection of remedies, and an enormously more extensive range of remedies from which to select.

"The trained radiesthetic sense, aided by a suitable instrument, can be of great assistance in remedy selection, but that is not the subject of this article, which is concerned with the remedies themselves.

"For the practitioner to be prepared to meet any requirement immediately would necessitate an enormous stock of remedies, each in a range of potencies. This would entail extensive storage space, and at present prices, a not inconsiderable capital investment.

"I cannot claim that the foregoing considerations resulted in my searching for methods of preparing Homoeopathic remedies, other than the customary series of alternating succussions and dilutions: but having stumbled upon an alternative method, I readily recognised its potential.

"This alternative method, which I have called Magneto-geometric potency preparation" came about in the following manner:-

"Radiesthetists frequently use a 100 cm. rule, along which to measure the "potency energy" of a sample of a remedy. With the sample located at the "zero" end of the rule, they move the

*Journal Research Society for Natural Theraputics

pendulum along the rule from left to right, noting the point at which the pendulum swings exactly at right angles to the rule. This point indicates a relative potency energy.

"It occurred to me that the point of balance thus detected is, in fact, the "boundary" between the remedy's local energy field, and a component of the earth's magnetic field, and this view was to some extent corroborated by the observation that measurements made with the rule differently orientated in relation to the terrestial field yielded different balance points.

"This lead to a series of measurements being made in respect of several different remedies, using the remedy vial as the central point, and finding the balance point along the rule, with it pointing in turn to each of the Cardinal and half Cardinal points of the compass. The results of these measurements were then plotted on polar graph paper, and the adjacent points joined by

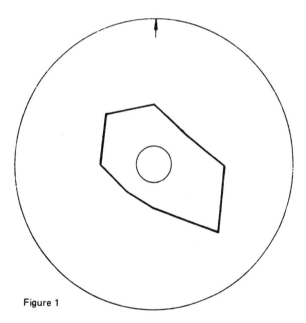

Figure 1

Circular Potency Simulator card representing
Argentum Nitricum

straight lines to form a geometric pattern related to each remedy. Each point was found to be solely related to one remedy.

"If the interaction of the remedy's energy field with the earth's field resulted in a pattern related to the remedy, it seemed not unlikely that the interaction of the earth's field and the pattern could be used to create a replica of the remedy, and experiments proved this to be the case.

"An interesting point then discovered was that the alignment of the pattern with the orientation in which it had been drawn resulted in the replica being of a very high potency (theoretically, infinite potency), whilst the greater the degree of misalignment the lower the potency replicated. From this, a scale was developed, against which to set the pattern to the required potency. At that time – 1966 – a number of patterns related to remedies were prepared, each drawn on a circular disc orientated North – South, and a few experimental instruments were constructed. The remedy discs were similar to those depicted as Figure 1, and the "instrument" approximately as shown in Figure 2.

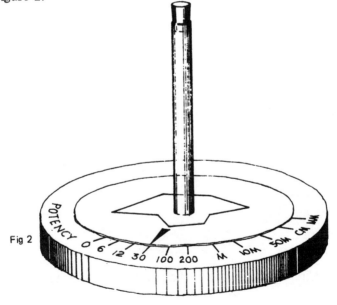

Fig 2

The original potency simulator "instrument."

"Tests made with a number of remedies prepared in this manner indicated them to be radiesthetically matched with conventionally prepared remedies: and their effects upon those taking them appeared to be similar: and, in fact, they were encouraging enough to stimulate the consideration of a less crude instrument. Amongst a number of obvious shortcomings in the initial design, it seemed imperative that the following should be eliminated:-

(a) circular remedy cards would be costly to produce, inconvenient to store, and would restrict the diameter of the vial used which must be the same as the hole in the card.

(b) the use of the earth's field as an energiser meant that the instrument must be correctly orientated, for were it misorientated, it would yield a potency other than that indicated on the scale.

To overcome the former, experiments were undertaken to discover whether the influence of the energised pattern could be guided along a wire from the centre of the drawing to the base of a cylindrical container into which a vial could be placed. These experiments confirmed that this could be done, with the result that the pattern could be located vertically, and thus be removed from the relevant effects of the earth's field.

"Further experiments showed that the earth's field could be replaced by that of a small permanent magnet: and hence it became possible to enclose the instrument in a suitable case. During the investigations, it had been discovered that a card bearing a circle, magnetically energised, would erase the pattern from a potentised medium placed within the circle: and also that it would erase the potency energy from a conventionally prepared Homoeopathic remedy. The potency could be restored to the conventionally prepared remedy by succussion, without the addition of further substance: whereas all record of the remedy was erased from a magneto-geometrically prepared remedy. It was therefore decided to incorporate a "neutraliser" in the form of a magnetically energised circle, which could be switched to the base of the cylindrical vial container, which became known as the "well".

"Energised by a permanent magnet, the vertically located pattern resulted in the production of energy of "infinite potency", which, due to circuit losses, was reduced to slightly above

10MM. From this varying amounts of energy had to be drawn off, to yield the required potency at the base of the instrument's well.

"It was found that this control-of potency could be achieved by a potential divider, for which purpose an ordinary radio potentiometer is suitable. The latter could be set against a scale marked with the customarily used potencies − or, of course, at any point between them: and to just the degree that accuracy of potencies is important, this facility for selecting intermediate potencies by interpolation is valuable.

"The gradations of the potency scale were set up to correspond with averages of stated potencies of new, previously unopened, remedies from various Homoeopathic chemists.

"The sizes of division on the scale furnish an indication of the relative potency energy field of the various potencies: whereas the numbers by which they are customarily described merely indicate the number of stages of dilution and succussion involved

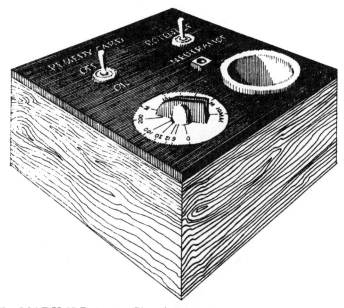

The MARK II Potency Simulator

in their preparation.

"Thus, the energy field of a 200C is only about twice that of a 30C, and that of a 1M is about twice that of a 100C.

"The Mark I potency simulator, contained in a wooden case, was constructed to incorporate the results of the foregoing researchers, and a number of these were made and tested over a period of two years before being superceded by the first "production model", – the Mark II, – which was similar, except that the case was entirely of perspex.

"It should be explained that the term "potency simulator" rather than "potentiser" or "potency maker" was adopted, because, whilst the instruments prepared remedies which apparently exerted exactly the same effect upon a patient as did their conventionally prepared counterparts, it was not then known whether any difference beyond the method of preparation, did, in fact, exist.

"Interest in this model, largely from overseas, lead to the design of a compact version – the Mark III – which has the advantage of a larger detachable well, for which it uses a standard size vial of 88 cc capacity, thus enabling stocks of remedies to be prepared in the containers in which they are to be stored, and of the absence of all switching, the instrument being so designed that it "potentises" whenever there is a remedy card in the slot, and "neutralises" if there is no card in the slot.

"Whilst the instruments were undergoing development, so too were the remedy patterns. The original circular design had been superceded by rectangular cards which fitted into a slot in the top of the instrument, and bore the remedy pattern in an improved form. The transition from the earlier to the later forms occurred when it was discovered that the patterns could be drawn using arbitrary orientations of the rule as already described, or by selecting a fixed point on the rule and slowly rotating it degree by degree, and marking the orientations at which the pendulum swings at right angles to the rule over the selected point. The latter proved to be the more convenient method.

"Furthermore it was found that the lines joining the points on the original patterns were unnecessary, the points themselves being the operative factors. Data for cards is obtained radiesthetically, using the constant formula:- "The ascending series of angles, each expressing to the nearest whole degree of arc, between the vertical radius representing no degrees from the centre of the potency simulator diagram, which solely represents . . . . . . (name of remedy), in such a way that a perfect potency of it may be prepared in the potency simulator for which the card is designed".

"To this formula, expressed as a symbol, the brain will respond in the same way as it responds to other symbols which instruct it how to think about a given subject, as, for example, a "£" sign, which tells the reader how to regard the numeral which follows it. When the reader sees "£5", he will hardly be aware of the "£" sign, which nevertheless controls the context in which he considers the "5".

"Informative symbols of this type can be described as "operators", and the formula for finding the data for simulator cards, has been crystallised into an operator, to ensure that whilst dowsing for the cards' data, the dowser's thoughts are influenced only by the precise definition of the data he requires.

"Data having been obtained, a master card is drawn, using the degree marks of a much larger circle than those printed on the production cards, in order to produce greater accuracy. The production cards are then printed photographically from the master card.

Agraphis Nutans

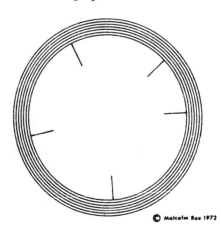

© Malcolm Rae 1972

"Each card may require up to 6 partial radii, and it is interesting to note that combinations of 6 radii drawn to an accuracy of 1 degree of arc, amount to 467,916,713,911,200 — so there is no liklihood of shortage of representation space.

"More elaborate models of the simulator have developed, but with one exception, which will be described later, they all employ the same principle. The information which has lead to these instruments does not depend upon the application of any theoretical knowledge previously known to the writer — and in an attempt to make the process by which the remedies are prepared seem a little less "improbable" the following model of how it *might* operate, is offered:-

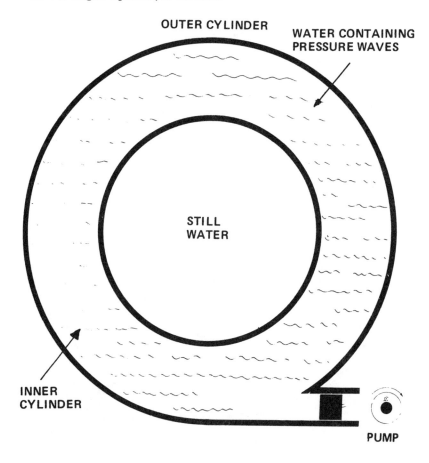

"The process depends primarily upon the capacity of water to accept and convey any magnetically energised pattern which is appropriately applied to it. This peculiarity enables water to be "potentised" — or charged — from a geometric pattern representing any remedy, and to become the equivalent of a "potency" of that remedy.

"An interesting observation is that any substance can be charged with its own potency energy, but water, alone, can be charged with the potency energy of any other substance.

"The best analogy available is this:-

(1)   Imagine a plan view of two concentric cylindrical open-topped tanks each almost full of water. Imagine that the

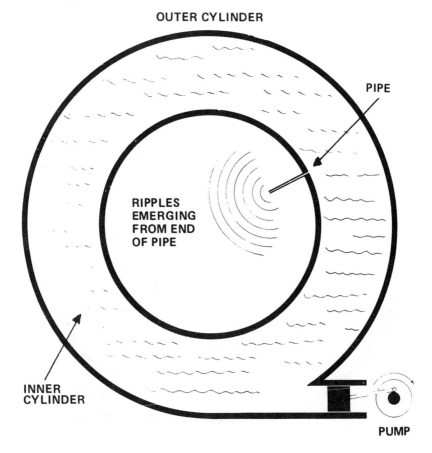

outer tank has entering it a pipe from a pump which rhythmically increases and decreases the pressure inside it. Under such circumstances, the water in the outer tank will be disturbed by pressure waves, from which the water in the inner tank will be screened by its cylindrical construction.

(2)   Now imagine a short length of pipe extending towards the centre of the inner tank from a hole in its side. From the inner end of the pipe, ripples will be formed.

(3)   Add a second length of pipe from another hole in the side of the inner tank, and ripples will emerge from it, to mingle with those from the first pipe, forming an interference pattern.

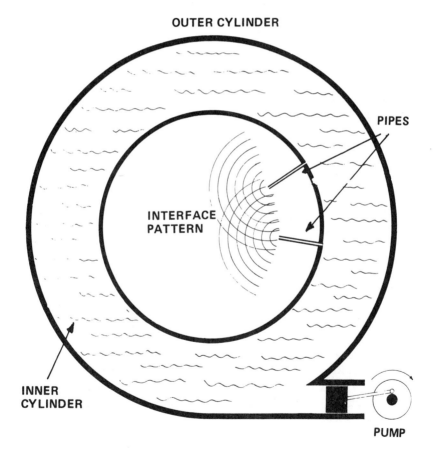

OUTER CYLINDER

PIPES

INTERFACE
PATTERN

INNER
CYLINDER

PUMP

"In the foregoing analogy, the pulsating water in the outer tank represents the pulsations attributed to the magnet, and the inner tank and pipes represent the simulator card, on which printed lines are able to carry the magnetic pulsations.

"The interference pattern is not affected by size, but is dependent solely upon proportion: and it may be compressed into a connection from a point at or near its centre, and lead to a circular disc, wherein it expands to cover the area of the disc. A vial of water, standing on the disc, will become charged with the pattern of the card – as long as the vial holding the water is cylindrical in shape. The pattern within the circle is a function of the following factors:-

(1) The nature of the vibrations applied to it.
(2) The number of partial radii.
(3) The relative lengths of the partial radii.
(4) The angular distance apart of the partial radii.

"However, since the magnetic vibrations employed are a facet of the Universe, they may be regarded as constant, and by making all the partial radii the same length, the pattern becomes dependant only upon the number of partial radii, and the angular distance between them.

"Excluding surgery, manipulation, and methods involving direct adjustment of the patient's physical body, there appear to be no more than two basic ways in which a therapist can influence him. He can introduce into the patient coded instructions designed to remind him what to do to remedy his disorders (which would include all oral remedies other than food supplements), and he can provide him with the material substances required by his organism to fulfil those instructions. All Homoeopathic remedies, however prepared, above about 12C potency, and all magneto-geometrically prepared remedies, regardless of potency, are solely coded message bearers, and nothing else. They do not contain the material, but only the information pattern of the substance they represent.

"It must be stressed that exact equivalents of conventionally made Homoeopathic remedies below 12C, or of tissue salts, cannot be made by magneto geometry: for whilst it can replicate the thought which defines the material, it cannot create the material.

"In practice, it appears to be the "message" only which is required for most administrations of even low potency preparations – but the limitation must not be overlooked.

"Outside of that limitation, magneto-geometric preparation has a number of advantages, and no disadvantages known to me. Amongst the advantages are the following:-

(1) Remedies prepared by magneto-geometry are consistently as accurate as the standard to which the cards are drawn. They cannot vary due to variations in mother tinctures. Nor can they be influenced by the substance of the containers in which they were potentised.

(2) Regardless of the potency required, only one process is needed, occupying a maximum of 6 minutes. This removes all liability of error which might occur in the long sequence of processes, and it enables high potencies of new remedies to be prepared in minutes.

(3) To prepare remedies, such as Oxygen M, which would be difficult if not impossible to prepare by succussion-dilution, is no problem. Hence the range of remedies available to the Homoeopath has been greatly extended by the development of the magneto-geometric method.

(4) The ability to prepare a remedy within minutes relieves the practitioner of the need to carry large stocks, and enables him to provide a remedy or potency which he does not have in stock, without having to order it and await its arrival. Moreover, instruments are small enough for a visiting doctor to carry one, together with a suitable selection of cards, on his rounds.

(5) The cost of each card, from which an unlimited quantity of the remedy, in any potency, may be prepared, is only about the same as the cost of the smallest vial of a manufactured remedy.

(6) The list of Homoeopathic remedies for which cards are available exceeds 2,000, and continues to increase in response to requests for remedies not yet listed.

Consideration of these advantages focusses the attention upon two serious weaknesses in the descriptions applied to Homoeopathic preparations. These are:-

(1) As previously observed, the number used to describe the

potency of a preparation does not describe the preparation itself, but relates only to the number of stages of succussion to which it has been subjected, and the degree of dilution at each stage. It is, then, little wonder that radiesthetically competent Homoeopaths have not infrequently observed differences between remedies bearing the same description, from different manufacturers — for the actual potency is dependent upon many factors, amongst which are:-

(a)　The number of stages of succussion and dilution.

(b)　The number of succussions per stage.

(c)　The degree of dilution per stage, which is normally standardised to one in ten parts or to one in one hundred.

(d)　The violence of the impact of each succussion.

(e)　The orientation of travel prior to that impact.

(f)　The length of travel prior to that impact.

There are probably other factors, but the foregoing are enough to render it obvious, that unless all were standardised throughout all manufacturers, differences in products would surely occur.

(2)　The second weakness to which I would refer is an overlooked factor which might be described as "the quality of the remedy", and the most suitable analogy by which to illustrate it is electrical. Two definitions normally applied to a Homoeopathic remedy are:-

(a)　The substance from which it is prepared, which might be called its "characteristic".

(b)　Its potency, which might be regarded as its "voltage". The "characteristic" of a car battery could be described as "direct current electro motive force", and its voltage would probably be nominally twelve measured when the battery is not connected to a circuit which is drawing power from it. However, the time throughout which a battery will remain at twelve volts when apparatus connected to it is drawing on its current, is called its capacity, and is expressed in ampere-hours. The number of ampere-hours available will depend on the size of the battery, and the amount of charge which it is holding. Together, these two factors might be termed its "quality". When an oral remedy is taken by a patient, it is similar to a little battery from which is drawn the patient's requirement. If the remedy is of poor quality, the patient's requirements soon discharges it, and renders it ineffectual. If it is of high quality, however, it will be better able to meet the patient's needs.

"The quality of a succussion-dilution prepared remedy is probably dependent upon the factors which I have enumerated, or at least upon some of them. Observation of Dr. Hahnemann's instructions produced a high quality remedy. The quality of a remedy may be measured radiesthetically, on a 100 cm. rule having a circular disc at the zero end. The remedy is placed upon the disc, and the extent of the energy field along the rule is measured with a pendulum. A magnet is brought close to the edge of the disc at the same instant that a stop watch is started, and the magnet will start to neutralise the remedy and reduce its field. A continuous check on the measurement along the rule is made, until it has reached exactly half its original measurement, at which times the watch is stopped. The time which has elapsed whilst the reduction in measurement has occurred may be regarded as the half life of the remedy under those circumstances, and the longer it is, the better is the remedy's quality.

"If standard comparative measurements are to be made in this matter, it is of course necessary to have the rule correctly orientated and remote from ferrous metal: it is necessary to use a standard size and material of disc, and it is necessary to use a standard magnet always identically placed: but Homoeopaths with radiesthetic sensitivity may make relative comparisons of remedies from their own stocks by the simple method I have outlined.

"Remedies prepared by the efficient application of magneto-geometry will be found to have about the highest "capacity" available, and may, amongst other positive characteristics, be expected to possess a commensurately long "shelf life" should the need arise to store them."

The article at this point deals briefly with another instrument called the Potency Preparer, which I would like to cover in a little more detail later on in the chapter; and then finishes with the following words:

"In conclusion, it should be stressed that whatever weaknesses exist in the theoretical understanding of magneto-geometric remedy preparation, the system has been well tried by many Homoeopaths. There are more than 1,000 instruments currently in use, in 23 different countries, and an ever-increasing demand for additions to the already 2,000 — strong card repertoire."

Like radionic instrumentation and rates, the ratio cards and the Simulator relate very directly to the various principles operating in the Universal Field of mind, and the energies present in that field. All esoteric teachings speak of the vital force or magnetic fluid that radiates from the sun and constitutes the life-essence of each of the seven planes. Blavatsky called it fohat, prana, electricity or magnetic fluid; Karl von Reichenbach referred to it as the odic force, John Keely the molecular ether or dynaspheric force, and in more recent times Dr. Wilhelm Reich rediscovered the life force and called it orgone energy. Basically these are all different names that have been attached to the one pervasive force that has been recognised by the ancient seers for thousands of years as the energy of matter. In radionics I believe that we are just touching on the borderlands where the relationship between prana and mind comes about, those like Keely, Von Reichenbach and Reich who pushed too far into this dangerous territory, met with incredible opposition, ridicule and persecution. Many see this phenomena as an act of the Establishment against anyone who delves into living forces. While this is probably true, it is my feeling that when a man like Keely can harness unlimited power out of thin air and drive a motor so fast that it almost tears loose from its base, or can cause an eight pound model of a zepplin to fly around a room, then he, like Wilhelm Reich who also discovered a 'motor force' in orgone has found something that in the wrong hands could be used to hold the world to ransom. Reich was so aware of this that he never committed his discovery to paper and the secret died with him in prison. Blavatsky said of Keely, that he was stopped from making any more headway in his discoveries by the Spiritual Hierarchy of our planet; the world and humanity are just not yet capable of dealing with such stupendous forces, and those who are successful in probing beyond certain limits will find that they run into a wall of resistance from every direction. The reason for this is given in *A Treatise on Cosmic Fire* by Alice

Bailey, and I think it worth outlining here because it brings in
once again the concept of the bridge that must be built by each
individual to link the lower and higher aspects of mind. Bailey
writes:

> The revelation of the close connection between mind and fohat or
> energy, or between thought power and electrical phenomena — the
> effect of fohatic impulse on matter — is fraught with peril, and the
> missing link (if so it might be termed) in the chain of reasoning from
> phenomena to its initiatory impulse, can only be safely imparted
> when the bridge between higher and lower mind, is adequately
> constructed. When the lower is under the control of the higher, or
> when the quaternary is merging into the triad, then man can be
> trusted with the remaining four fundamentals.

If you doubt that radionics is a healing art primarily concerned with the manipulation of the life-force by means of the
mind, then consider for one moment what happened to Dr.
Albert Abrams who was ceaselessly persecuted and vilified for
his discoveries which led to radionics as we know it today.
Consider too, the fate of Ruth Drown who in the seventh decade
of her life was imprisoned for her work in radionics. Even in
Britain where the climate of opinion is a little more tolerant,
George de la Warr was drawn into a court case that so depleted
his energy and funds that he was almost forced to desist from
the remarkable work he did in this field. By its very nature, the
life-force invokes a resistance against all those who would probe
its secrets. Such a path of discovery is not meant to be easy, and
secrets wrested from this aspect of nature are only obtained at
great cost to the personality or low-self, which in the final
analysis is of no account if a step closer to the Source of Truth
has been made by the individual concerned. I have always maintained that radionics is more than a healing art, for if one looks
beyond the phenomena it can clearly be discerned as a field of
human endeavour that will serve to build the individual and
group antahkarana. Radionics is a bridge between the physical
and subtle realms, between orthodox and spiritual medicine,
and thus its practitioners and pioneers are bridge builders be
they conscious of the fact or not. This has the profoundest of
implications for those who are prepared to look deeper into this
concept.

Well let us get back to the life-force in respect to potency simulation. The Simulator is a perspex box containing amongst other things a circular magnet, in effect it is an accumulator for the life-force. Much of Von Reichenbach's investigations into the odic force as he called it, revolved around the studies made by sensitives, many of them medical doctors, who could see the auric field of various objects including magnets. These people worked with Von Reichenbach to provide him with descriptions of the force and the way it behaved under various circumstances. They invariably describe the force field around a magnet as being surrounded by a blue aura at the north end and a yellowish-red at the south, between were greens, violets and indigos all flickering and moving like flames across the surface of the metal. He found too that the odylic force could be conducted along wire very easily. Copper wire conducts heat for only a few inches, Reichenbach's sensitives could see the activity of the life-force at a distance of seventy feet along the same wire, making it appear to glow in the darkness. Malcolm Rae discovered in effect, the same phenomena occured during his experimental work that led to the construction of the MARK I Potency Simulator. Sensitives could feel the effect of the odylic force for a distance of up to four hundred feet from a magnet, so in terms of the life-force the magnet carries an enormous radiatory power.

Reichenbach found also that odyle entered into the mass of any body it charged, but travelled slowly along a wire, taking some 20-40 seconds to traverse 50-60 yards. In the Simulator this effect is constant and the wire fully charged at all times. He also notes in his book on the odic force that it can be stimulated into action by an electrical impulse from a distance; a 2 inch spark for example, exciting a vivid current of odyle in a wire six and a half feet away.

Experiments were run that showed all solids and liquids can be charged with odyle, but he adds that this charge is not discernible to the sensitive for any longer than one hour. The work done in potency simulation and the results obtained from treatment with medicines made in this way clearly shows that the liquid or sac lac does retain the pattern that it is exposed to, so perhaps in this case the combination of odylic force, the magnetic force and the pattern have an effect that is longer lasting than simple exposure to the one force.

Reichenbach's sensitivities could very definitely identify water that had been exposed to odic forces, and also differentiate between those that had stood in moonlight and sunlight. Today in Russia a great deal of medical experimentation is going on in which three specialists Drs. Shevtsov, Tovstoles and Grebenschchikov are treating patients at the Kirov Military Academy with water that has been treated magnetically. Once considered a form of quackery, magnetized liquids are now proving very effective in the treatment of such diverse diseases as heart trouble, chronic bronchitis, liver and kidney problems and hypertension, and a whole new field of medicine known as Magneto-Biology has come into being.

Soviet researchers now believe that this kind of treatment has its primary influence upon the body through the hypothalamus, which from an esoteric point of view is an externalisation or aspect of the brow chakra that governs the pituitary. Curiously, a person with a highly active integrated functioning pituitary is inevitably referred to as having a 'magnetic personality'.

Treatment takes two forms; the magnetized water is either introduced into the urinary tract by means of a catheter or put into tea, coffee or soups which are ingested by the patients. The preparation of magnetically treated water is interesting in that the water never touches the magnets at any time. It is simply allowed to drip between the poles of two adjacent magnets, and collected in a container. To a sensitive the flames of odylic energy pour from the ends of a magnet; what is happening in these Russian experiments is fairly obvious, that the water is picking up the charge of the life-force as it falls between the magnets. In some instances the water is passed along a glass tube which must lengthen the time of exposure to the energy field, but to my knowledge there are no statistics to suggest that this creates a stronger form of medicine or that it gets better results.

From a potency simulation point of view these recent developments in Russia are encouraging in that with only one aspect of Magneto-Geometric principles, they are getting provable results. The Potency Simulator with its other aspects of geometric patterning and controlled potency must eventually be proved superior.

In order to round out this chapter let us return to the details of the various instruments that have been developed for potency simulation and preparation which can be used by any practitioner to prepare remedies, or as we shall see, for purposes of radionic treatments at a distance.

HOMOEOPATHIC POTENCY PREPARATION BY MAGNETICALLY ENERGISED GEOMETRIC PATTERNS

A. PRINCIPLE:
1. The specific characteristics of any substance may be expressed numerically as a group of ratios, or represented by a pattern geometrically expressing ratios.
2. The appropriate application of magnetism to a geometric expression of a substance creates an influence which will be recorded by water, whether free, or as a component of any other substance, which lies within that influence.
3. The appropriate application of magnetism to any substance will create an influence which will be recorded by water within that influence.
4. The water so influenced is the equivalent in its effect upon a living organism, of a conventionally prepared homoeopathic medicine.

B. APPLICATION OF PRINCIPLE TO INSTRUMENTS:-
1. Instruments designed to employ this principle have been in use for several years, and over 1,000 are currently in use.
2. A stock of some 3,000 geometric patterns, on cards measuring 75mm x 65mm, includes those representing almost every well-known homoeopathic medicine, and many hundreds of less-known remedies.
3. The basic structure of the instruments is a small box equipped with one or more slots into which remedy cards fit, one or more calibrated controls, on which the required potency(ies) is/are set, and a "well" into

which the phial containing the distilled water or other substance (usually sac lac) to be potentised, is placed.
4. Each instrument is also fitted with two sockets: one to accept a single plug enabling it to be connected to a radionic projector of suitable design; and the other to accept a jack plug connected to a suitable pulse generator (interrupter) to convert the instrument into a radionic projector.

C. VARIANTS OF POTENCY SIMULATOR:-
1. The following variants are available:-
   (i) Mark III Potency Simulator operating from cards. (Paragraph G).
   (ii) Extended-Range Potency Simulator operating from cards. (Paragraph H).
   (iii) Extended-Range 4 section Multiple Remedy Potency Simulator operating from cards. (Paragraph J).
   (iv) Twin Well Magnetic Homoeopathic Potency Preparer operating from substance or homoeopathic potency.
2. In the following pages, each instrument will be described in detail, and instructions given for its use.

D. COMMON FACTORS IN DESIGN OF INSTRUMENTS:-
1. All instruments have been designed to be as simple as possible.
2. All instruments are constructed by a fully qualified (M.B.H.I.) instrument maker, and every effort has been made to ensure that no fault can develop in them.
3. All instruments are entirely magnetically energised, requiring neither mains connections nor batteries to prepare homoeopathic remedies.
4. They are independent of the earth's magnetic field and need no special orientation.
5. All card-operated instruments have built-in neutralisation circuits which operate automatically when there is no card in the slot, to erase all characteristics from no longer wanted preparations, leaving them clear to

accept further potentisation.

6. Since the potency by which a homoeopathic remedy is described indicates only the number of stages of succussion to which it has been subjected, and the degree of dilution at each stage, it cannot be regarded as a standard measurement, and indeed samples of the same potency of the same remedy from different manufacturing chemists frequently vary greatly.

7. Until there is a standard against which to calibrate instruments (and such a standard would be necessarily complex) the only workable method is to match the instruments to the average of a number of samples of different remedies rated by their manufacturers at the same potency. This is what has been done.

E. ADVANTAGES OF MAGNETO-GEOMETRIC POTENCY PREPARATION:-

This method of preparing remedies is believed to possess the following advantages:-

1. Consistency of remedies:- all remedies made in these instruments from any given card have identical characteristics.

2. Purity:-
   (i) The geometric figure on the card is drawn to represent the remedy in its perfect state: it cannot become contaminated during manufacture, by the addition of traces of substances from which manufacturing apparatus is constructed.
   (ii) A card drawn to represent a vegetable remedy in its perfect state will exclude the effects of variations in the soil, and of other conditions of growth.
   (iii) Phials may be re-used after washing and neutralisation.

3. Speed:-
   (i) It requires no longer to make a remedy of 10MM potency than to make one of 12C.
   (ii) The practitioner may carry the instrument and a selection of remedy cards when visiting patients,

and thus be enabled to prepare remedies immediately, on the spot.

4. Economy:-
    (i) Because any potency of any remedy may be prepared within minutes, there is no reason for the practitioner to hold a large and comprehensive stock representing considerable frozen capital.
    (ii) Unwanted remedies resulting from over production may be reduced to sac lac for further use.

5. Versatility:-
    A simulator card may be prepared for any substance or concept that can be exactly defined. Hence potencies may be made to represent gases and other unhandleable substances, thus greatly extending the possible range of remedies.

F. ADVANTAGES OF THE CARD SYSTEM:-
    1. As stated under "PRINCIPLE" it is possible to express the potency characteristics of substance numerically as well as geometrically, and it is therefore possible to construct an instrument equipped with a number of calibrated dials on which could be set the numerical constants of the substance from which a potency is required.

        It is believed, however, that an instrument using cards rather than numbered dials possesses the following advantages, and no disadvantages:-
    (a) (i) Remedies prepared from cards are consistently as accurate as the standard to which the cards are drawn: whereas, due to parallax (the effect of the angle from which the dial setting is viewed), thickness of calibrations, etc., numerical settings would vary from time to time, and from operator to operator.
        (ii) The cards prepared for use with the Rae instruments are printed reproductions of masters which are extremely accurately drawn.
    (b) (i) The probability of preparing a potency from the

wrong card, located in the instrument with the name facing the operator, is negligible.

(ii) The probability of an error occurring during the sequence of looking up the numerical representation of a remedy and setting it on a series of dials is very much greater.

(c) Because panels carrying several numerically calibrated dials are not required, it has been possible to make the Rae instruments more compact, and much simpler than any instrument using numerical settings. They are, therefore, cheaper to produce and contain virtually nothing which could become faulty.

G. THE MARK III POTENCY SIMULATOR: this is the original production model, only marketed after 4 years testing by a number of homoeopaths.

INSTRUCTIONS – MARK III POTENCY SIMULATOR:-
1. To Prepare a Potency:-
   (It is imperative that the following sequence of operations is observed.)
(i) With the instrument positioned with the slot at the end furthest from the operator, insert the card for the required remedy in the slot, with the name upwards and facing the operator.
(ii) Set the pointer of the potency control to the required potency.
(iii) Place the medium to be potentised either directly in the well of the instrument, or in a previously neutralised phial in the well of the instrument. *IMPORTANT:* only cylindrical phials should be used.
(iv) If sac lac is the medium to be potentised, the pilules should be moistened prior to placing them in the simulator well. This is because the potentising process depends upon the presence of moisture in the medium to be potentised and although sac lac pilules usually contain some water, it is advisable to moisten them sufficiently for them to appear shiny, but not to cause them to start dissolving.

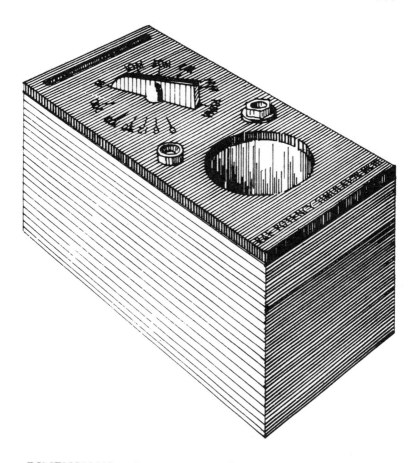

DIMENSIONS: Instrument: Overall length   152mm
                               Overall breadth   80mm
                               Overall height   85mm
              Well: Internal diameter 48mm
                               Internal depth   62mm
                               Internal capacity 112cc
              Total weight: 625gms

Because it has a more rapid evaporation rate than water, it is preferable to moisten with 30% (or thereabouts) alcohol.

D.R.—5

Gin or Vodka will meet this requirement without discolouring the sac lac.

For small quantities of pilules, it is convenient to use a short length of wire, which when dipped into the liquid used and then withdrawn, will form a small globule on its end. The volume of the globule depends upon the thickness of the wire and the depth to which it is lowered in the liquid.

For larger quantities of pilules, a dropping bottle is more suitable.

In either case the pilules should be thoroughly shaken after the liquid has been added, in order to spread it as evenly as possible over their surfaces.

(v)   Leave the medium in the well for a minimum of one minute if water is being potentised, and for a minimum of six minutes if sac lac is the medium.

(vi) The medium is fully potentised on termination of these times, and will not be affected by additional time in the instrument.

IMPORTANT: The potentised medium must be removed from the instrument before the remedy card is removed — otherwise the medium will be subjected to neutralisation.

2.   To Neutralise a Potency:-

(i)   Ensure that no remedy card is in the slot.

(ii) Set the potency control at 10MM.

(iii) Place the medium to be neutralised either directly in the well of the instrument, or in a phial in the well of the instrument. *IMPORTANT:* only cylindrical phials should be used.

(iv) Leave for a minimum of one minute if water, and a minimum of six minutes if sac lac.

(v)   The medium will then be neutral and ready to accept a further potentisation.

H.   THE EXTENDED RANGE POTENCY SIMULATOR: although a magneto-geometrically prepared remedy of potency below 12C does not exactly match its succussion-dilution prepared namesake, insofar as the former contains no material, whilst the latter contains traces of material, the experience of many users has proved low-potency magneto-geometrically prepared remedies to be effective. This variant was first designed in response to a request from Mark L. Gallert — author of *New Light on Theraputic Energies*, for an instrument in which the low potencies could be set more accurately than on the Mark III, of which the potency scale is unavoidably "bunched" below 12C. The Extended Range Potency Simulator employs a digital dial, calibrated from "000" to "1000" (though the "1" of the "1000" position does not appear on the dial), to provide a scale length approximately 12 times the length of that of the Mark III.

Since it is not possible to calibrate this type of dial directly in potencies, a conversion graph is necessary.

INSTRUCTIONS — THE EXTENDED RANGE POTENCY SIMULATOR:-

All instructions for the Extended Range Potency Simulator are identical with those for the Mark III with the exception of (ii).

Setting the required potency on the Extended Range Potency Simulator is achieved as follows:-

(i) Select the graph down the right-hand side of which the required potency appears.

(ii) Locate the required potency and follow the horizontal line from it to the left until it meets the curve of the graph.

(iii) From the point where it meets the curve of the graph, follow the vertical line down the scale along the bottom edge of the graph, and read off the instrument's dial setting.

(iv) On graph "A", range 1x to 12x, each small division along the base line represents 5°.
On graph "B", range 1c to 1M, each small division along the base line represents 10°.

(v) A small lever projecting from the front edge of the dial will lock the setting at any number. (See sketch.)

(vi) It is important to avoid forcing the dial beyond either the maximum or the minimum settings; or trying to turn the knob when the lock has been applied, as the mechanism may be damaged by so doing.

THE EXTENDED RANGE POTENCY SIMULATOR

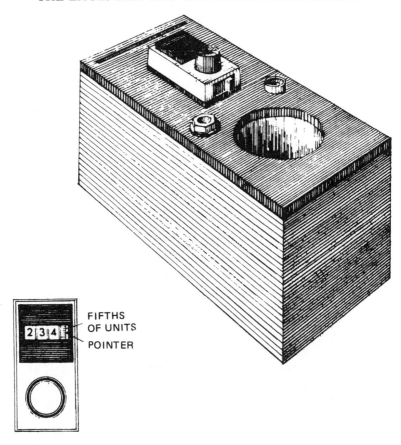

FIFTHS
OF UNITS
POINTER

UNLOCK   LOCK

DETAIL of DIGITAL DIAL

DIMENSIONS:	Instrument:	Overall length	152mm
		Overall breadth	80mm
		Overall height	90mm
	Well:	Internal diameter	48mm
		Internal depth	62mm
		Internal capacity	112cc
	Total weight:		625gms

J. THE EXTENDED RANGE 4-SECTION MULTIPLE RE-
MEDY POTENCY SIMULATOR:

It is not possible to prepare a multiple remedy consisting
of more than one component by potentising the medium
with the card for each component in turn, because each
potentisation partially erases the effects of its predecessors.
It can be done by potentising an equal volume of water
with the card for each component of the remedy and
mixing the results.

However, this is a time-consuming process, and the 4-section
Multiple Simulator was designed to solve the problem. It
can prepare a remedy with one, two, three or four components in one operation, with each component at the same
or different potencies.

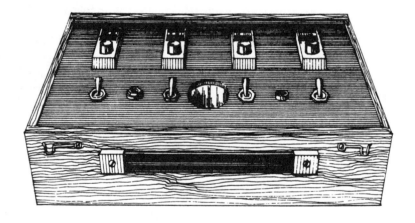

DIMENSIONS: Instrument: Overall length 340mm
Overall breadth 178mm
Overall height 100mm
Well: Internal diameter 48mm
Internal depth 62mm
Total weight: 2438gms

INSTRUCTIONS – THE EXTENDED RANGE 4-SECTION POTENCY SIMULATOR.

This instrument is operated in exactly the same way as the Extended Range Potency Simulator.

(i)   Single remedies may be prepared in the instrument by having all but one of the switches in the "OFF" position (ie. switch lever pointing towards the digital dial), setting the required potency, and inserting the remedy card in the section that is "ON" (ie. switch lever pointing away from the digital dial).

(ii) Multiple remedies consisting of up to four components may be prepared by inserting a card for each component in the slot of each section, setting the potency dial of each setting the potency dial of each section to the required potency, and the switch for each section that is in use at the "ON" position.

IMPORTANT: It is essential that switches for all sections not in use are set at "OFF".

The following instrument is distinctly different from the Potency Simulators in that it works to transfer a healing influence or quality from an original substance to a carrier substance such as sac lac or water.

K.   THE RAE MAGNETIC HOMOEOPATHIC POTENCY PRE-PARER

This instrument differs from those previously described, and is, in fact, complementary to them, its purpose being to prepare, in a single operation, without succussion, dilution, mechanical agitation, or the application of any external of energy, the following:-

(i)   any homoeopathic potency from a sample of any substance or combination of substances.

(ii) any homoeopathic potency from any other homoeopathic potency of the same substance.

THE RAE MAGNETIC HOMOEOPATHIC POTENCY PREPARER

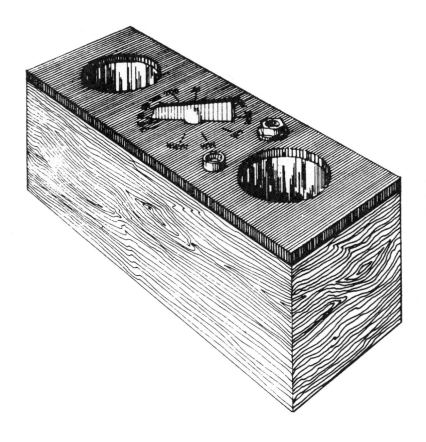

DIMENSIONS: Intrusment: Overal length   227mm
                               Overall breadth   94mm
                               Overall height   90mm
              Wells (each):   Internal diameter   48mm
                               Internal depth   62mm
                               Internal capacity 112cc
              Total weight: 790gms

INSTRUCTIONS – THE RAE MAGNETIC HOMOEOPATHIC POTENCY PREPARER

IT IS IMPERATIVE THAT THE FOLLOWING SEQUENCE OF OPERATIONS IS OBSERVED:-

1. To prepare a potency from a sample of any substance:-
(a) Place the sample in the "input well", in a cylindrical phial.
(b) Set the potency control to the desired potency.
(c) Place the medium to be potentised (distilled water, moistened sac lac, or acqueous cream, etc) in the "output well", in a cylindrical phial of the same substance as that used in the "input well". (i.e. Plastic in both, glass in both, etc).
(d) Leave for a minimum of 10 minutes. (Time in excess of ten minutes has no additional effect.)
(e) Remove the potentised medium from the "output well".
(f) Remove the sample from the "input well".
2. To prepare a potency from any other potency of the same substance:-
    Place the existing potency in the "input well", and follow the sequence 1. (a) to 1. (f) above.
    The potency to be prepared may be higher or lower than that of the existing potency.
3.
(a) In neither case is the sample destroyed by the process but it is raised to a very high potency (above 10MM), and should not, therefore, be held in the hand for more than a few seconds.
(b) This does not render it unsuitable for use in the preparation of further potencies, *but it must not be subsequently administered orally in the belief that it is unchanged.*
(c) Should it be desired to de-potentise a sample of *substance*, however, this may be done by allowing it to remain in the "output well", with the "input well" empty of everything including the cylindrical plastic phial, and the potency control set at 10MM, for a minimum of ten minutes.
4. It is, of course, necessary to sterilize the "input" phial immediately after it has contained any infectious or potentially infectious material.

SPECIAL APPLICATIONS:

Since the instrument prepares a potency of every aspect of the contents of the "input" phial, it is especially suitable for the preparation of:-

(i) Nosodes from patients' blood, urine, sputum, etc.
(ii) Individualistic remedies sometimes required in treating allergies, such as hair from a particular animal: pollen from a particular variety of flower: foodstuffs, etc.
(iii) Potencies of gems, where representation of the theraputic characteristic extends beyond the chemical composition.
(iv) Potencies of mixtures of substances. (But not potencies of mixtures of different potencies, because the components would all be reduced or expanded to the same potency.)

The details and instructions for use of the Magneto-Geometric Analyser, the various Magneto-Geometric Potency Simulators and the Potency Preparer, have been included because this book is designed to serve as a manual for practitioners which can be referred to on a day to day basis during practice. This will become even more evident in the latter sections and chapters of the book where many points will be touched upon relative to the practical aspects of treating by radionics.

It has been mentioned that the Potency Simulator can be used as a radionic treatment instrument if linked to an interrupter, so that radionics can be broadcast to the patient at a distance. For example, if a patient has earache and Belladonna is indicated, then the patient's sample can be put in the well of the instrument, the potency of remedy set on the indicator and the interrupter turned on, this will effectively beam the pattern of Belladonna to the patient. The simulator has of course been used for the treatment of soil and plants and in one instance experiments were carried out by a medical mining officer in South Africa who was concerned with the high density of anopheline mosquitos in the area, using such a method of broadcasting. His telegram to Malcolm Rae from Pretoria in April 1975 read:

ANOP GAMBIA EXPOSURE EIGHTEEN DAYS TO PATTERN –
LAST LARVAE COUNT NIL FROM WORST INFECTED AREAS –
THANKS TO YOU – AS ABOVE SO BELOW . . . . . SEELOS

The anopheline mosquito carries malarial parasites known as

plasmodia, which it transmits to the bloodstream of man when the skin is pierced as it bites its victim. No doubt this medical officer was delighted to have found a method of getting rid of the offending mosquitos and thus cutting back the chances of the mining staff from contracting malaria, without having to saturate the area with DDT or other pesticides.

There can be no doubt from the reams of correspondence I have seen, that radionic instrumentation based on magneto-geometric principles can be used in a wide variety of situations and for an equally varied number of purposes. Certainly they will meet the requirements of any busy and conscientious practitioner, no matter in what area of the healing arts his discipline lies.

SECTION THREE

Occult Pathology

The main reason for the failure of modern medical science is that it is dealing with results and not causes. For many centuries the real nature of disease has been masked by materialism, and thus disease itself has been given every opportunity of extending its ravages, since it is not attacked at its origin. The situation is like to an enemy strongly fortified in the hills, continually waging guerilla warfare in the country around, while the people, ignoring the fortified garrison, content themselves with repairing damaged houses and burying the dead, which are the result of the raids of the marauders. So, generally speaking, is the situation in medicine today; nothing more than the patching up of those attacked and the burying of those who are slain, without a thought being given to the real stronghold.

Disease will never be cured or eradicated by present materialistic methods, for the simple reason that disease in its origin is not material.

Edward Bach, M.B., B.S., D.P.H.

CHAPTER EIGHT

The Conflict between Energies and Force

*Disease is a form of active energy, demonstrating in
forces which destroy or produce death. Therefore, if
our basic premise is correct, disease is also a form of
divine expression, for what we know to be evil is also
the reverse side of that which we call good.*
                    Esoteric Healing — Alice A. Bailey

To the orthodox medical practitioner, disease is seen as a
definite morbid process which gives rise to a number of symptoms which are in the main considered to be triggered off by a
variety of physical agents such as bacteria or virus. The persistent
ability of the latter to constantly adapt itself and modify its
structure, and thus frustrate the efforts of medical science to
bring it to heel, have caused it to become the butt and blame for
the endless minor and mysterious abberations to health that
patients present in consulting rooms all over the world. If it's
non-specific it must be a virus going around, and the patient is
told there's a lot of it about, whatever it is, and they are ordered
to rest and take this or that latest wonder nostrum from the drug

houses. The fact that over twenty five per cent of all hospital beds are filled as the result of iatrogenic, that is doctor caused disease, is no deterrent to this concept of disease and the treatment it should. by today's chemotheraputic standards receive. Even something as recognizably unphysical as general nervous tension and anxiety is greeted in the main by a standing order at the chemists for as many as 500 tablets of standard tranquilizers or anti-depressants. The pollution unleashed into the bodies of people under the guise of medical practice has reached almost equal proportions to the pollution of the earth itself by the same drug companies. When I see six year olds addicted to tranquilizers and their mothers drugged up to the eyebrows, and arthritics hallucinating as the result of prescribed drugs, then it would seem to me that all is not well in the world of medicine and that the physicality of its approach to the problems of disease seriously needs reviewing, particularly in the light of spiritual science and the alternative approaches to healing.

While almost any alternative medicine practitioner would agree that bacterial and viral infections are a demonstrable aspect of many disease conditions, they would in the main be inclined to argue that these only appear in sufficient numbers to become harmful when the soil of the body in which they plant themselves is in a poor condition and receptive to their advances. In other words bacteria and virus are not a primary cause of disease, but an effect, which when it becomes strongly established appears to be a cause. It is the cause of disease that concerns radionic practitioners and the whole procedure of a health analysis is to determine the basic causative factor behind any set of symptoms. In most cases the cause lies on subtle levels and can only be read in terms of energy imbalance which distort the various fields or vehicles of the patient. Of course we are dealing with subjective factors which are not seen to be scientifically provable, nevertheless treatment based on such findings can be dramatically effective.

It is only natural that the physical body with its symptom patterns, crowds to the forefront of our consciousness, but it must be understood that the physical body, and to a very great extent the etheric body, only mirror the problems that lie on the astral and mental levels of consciousness. If this is true then disease is not physical in nature at all, but can be only understood in terms of energy and force.

In *Esoteric Healing* by Alice Bailey a series of laws that concern the true healer are outlined. The fifth law gives the basic causes of disease, and I will repeat it here, adding in parenthesis my interpretation of the symbolic wording in an attempt to clarify the meaning. It reads:

> There is naught but energy, for God is Life. Two energies (those of Spirit and Matter) meet in man, but other five are present (those of the soul, and mental body, the astral body and the physical-etheric body, making four. The fifth is that energy comprising the sum total of the low-self). For each is to be found a central point of contact. The conflict of these energies with forces and of forces twixt themselves produce the bodily ills of man. The conflict of the first and second persists for ages until the mountain top is reached — the first great mountain top. The fight between the forces produces all disease, all ills and bodily pain which seek release in death. The two, the five and thus the seven plus that which they produce, possess the secret. This is the fifth law of healing within the world of form.

If that law seems to be rather abstruse, then know that it is deliberately worded in that way in order to hide its meaning. Dr. Edward Bach said exactly the same thing in his booklet *Heal Thyself* so I shall quote from him in order to clarify this point and hopefully at the same time simplify it.

> Disease is in essence the result of conflict between Soul and Mind, and will never be eradicated except by spiritual and mental effort.

and again:

> It is when our personalities are led astray from the path laid down by the Soul, either by our own worldly desires or by the persuasion of others, that a conflict arises.

What Dr. Bach and Alice Bailey are in essence saying is that when the outflow of energy from the soul meets the force fields of our various bodies, (which in themselves contain other pockets of force which we label with the words fear, resentment, hate, anger, jealousy, pride — all to be found in the astral and mental bodies, or miasms and toxins and other pollutants in the etheric body, we have a situation that creates friction, as soul energy strikes upon a focus of force in any vehicle. Friction eventually creates disease, which ultimately is precipitated upon the physical plane in the form of organic lesions or psychological disturbances. If soul energy flows unhindered through the personality and expresses itself as love and peace and harmony on the physical plane, then you'll have no disease. The power of life pours through us in all its perfection, why should it manifest as disease in individuals all over the world? Quite simply because on its way to expression it runs into blockages which impregnate it with patterns of distortion, we are not content, nor yet capable in most cases of letting the Universal Mind express Its purpose through us . . . we have plans of our own, the personality must assert itself and battle with life instead of allowing life to gently and effectively express Itself. This is what Dr. Bach calls the conflict between Soul and Mind and he is right because the esoteric teachings state quite definitely that the lower mind is the slayer of the Real. However it must have its way until the lower-self is a fully functioning integrated unit, which will be of use to the soul in its projected plan. Disease and suffering are just side effects that are ultimately left behind when the personality finally surrenders to the soul and the mountain top is reached.

Again and again one comes across the theme of conflict between the various energies and forces in man as a cause of disease. Ethel Belle Morrow in her book *The Unseen Link* writes:

As man thinks, he rules his body or allows his body to rule him. Through his own thoughts effects he brings himself disease and destruction, and the vicious circle continues; the ills and the sins of the body through reactions cause emotions, restraints, revolts, and distrust until the good man would do is overcome by the powers of the flesh. Thoughts become reflex-action, as do characteristics and bodily acquirements, and the flesh rules the mind through these as effects taking part in the cause.

and:

As man rules his mind he brings his body under subjection; from thoughts of being well comes a quota of power to counteract the powers which have controlled his body, as disease. Man's attitudes and experiences are reactions of thought, and are the effect of conflicting powers; by controlling these, man can make very extensive repairs.

and:

> Because man's magnetic field is continually in contact with other magnetic fields, where the actions of the positive and negative powers are attracting and repelling, man is often contaminated through the interchange of these powers, as germs of disease, plagues, or a subnormal physical field. Man needs to neutralize the powers within, that the surrounding powers through the One Power may be kept under subjection.

and:

> A lack of control in the body and in its field of magnetism is the cause of many accidents. If the body is controlled entirely, the feelings of pain, anger, anguish, hunger, heat and cold can be controlled, also loves, hates, desires, restraints, emotions, and attitudes which, unless controlled by the neutralization of thought powers that allow the flow of the One Power, will be detrimental to the mind as well as the body.

In Eastern medicine, particularly acupuncture, the entire basis of practice is posited upon the primordial powers of yin and yang. The balance of these opposites within the energy systems of man brings health, and excess or lack of one or the other expresses itself as disease. Health manifests when there is a unity of purpose between the soul and the personality, which has progressed to a state of surrender to the higher purpose. In *The Yellow Emperor's Classic of Internal Medicine* Ch'i Po in a dialogue with the Emperor says, "The utmost in the art of healing can be achieved when there is unity." The Emperor enquires, "What is meant by unity?" to which Ch'i Po answers:

> "When the minds of the people are closed and wisdom is locked out they remain tied to disease. Yet their feelings and desires should be investigated and made known, their wishes and ideas should be followed; and then it becomes apparent that those who have attained spirit and energy are flourishing and prosperous, while those perish who lose their spirit and energy."

Until the battle between the soul and its mechanism ends in the surrender of the lower to the higher, there will always be conflict between these dual forces. Time and experience become factors which eventually lead man out of this state, as he learns in each new crisis of consciousness to look towards the One Power and to follow with understanding that profound instruction to: 'Resist not evil'. An ancient aphorism carries the same message of surrender which leads man from darkness to light and from the ravages of disease to harmony. It goes:

Cease from thy doing. Walk not on the Path until thou hast learnt the art of standing still.
Study the spider, brother, entangled not in its web, as thou art today entangled in thine own.

The vehicles of our mind and emotion are filled with our plans and ambitions and hopes, our fears and desires, and all eventually, at least those that are not in accord with the inner purpose, have to be discarded, for as long as they remain there will be conflict and disease.

The following diagram may help to clarify this point regarding the clash between the energy of the soul and the forces contained in the subtle vehicles.

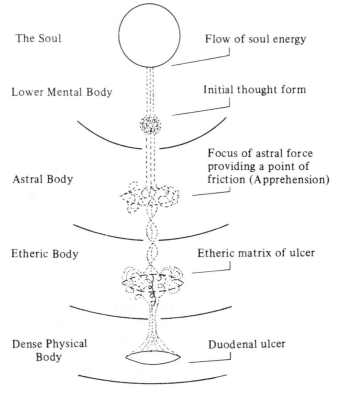

The Soul — Flow of soul energy

Lower Mental Body — Initial thought form

Astral Body — Focus of astral force providing a point of friction (Apprehension)

Etheric Body — Etheric matrix of ulcer

Dense Physical Body — Duodenal ulcer

The outflow of the soul's energy touches upon a thought form built by mental activity due to concern about some factor in the life experience of the individual. This reaches more powerful proportions as astral matter in the form of apprehension is added. When sufficiently potent, the energy of this astral form impresses its distortive pattern upon the etheric matrix and finally emerges in the physical body as an ulcer. All disease is a 'working outward' of distortions in energy flow upon the inner levels of consciousness.

The whole process of disease in the various bodies of man is at once an incredibly complex matter, and a very simple one. When faced with such a paradox it is difficult to know where to draw the line; too much detail only confuses, and too little does not meet the needs of the practitioner. Certainly there is not room in this book to cover the subject fully, so I will try to give what I consider to be certain basics which will provide the reader with a series of points of departure into areas that he or she can explore more fully as time passes. Above all in this, I want to maintain the theme of 'essential simplicity'.

Having given an airing to the fundamental concept that disease arises from the clash and distortions of energy flow in and through the subtle anatomy of man, we can now go ahead and take a look at certain aspects of this in more detail. For this purpose I think it will be best if I sub-divide the chapter into a series of headings to clearly delineate each area that we are going to cover.

DISEASE FACTORS IN THE MENTAL BODY

Christian Science and the adherents of the New Thought movement who do such excellent healing work, claim that disease has its origin in the mind of man. More esoteric schools of thought point out that man has yet to develop the mind more fully before it becomes a truly potent source of disease. They agree that the mind is involved to some extent but not to the exclusion of all else, and that because man is polarised or focussed primarily in his astral vehicle, it must inevitably be the prime source of trouble. Thoughts if clearly expressed and rightly motivated do not cause problems, the trouble arises as a thought is obliterated when stepped down to the level of the emotions. Here we come again to this matter of the right blend of kama-manas (feeling-mind) in which the astral and mental bodies are so closely blended as to make it difficult to distinguish thought from astral activity.

One of the fundamental laws of the Universal Mind is the law of cycles or periodicity which governs all the workings and processes of nature. Civilised man flouts this law which is given form on the mental plane, and in so doing may be said to create disease patterns at that level. No other creature breaks this law as does man. Consider for a moment his sleeping habits, going to bed late, often rising in a state of lethargy, rushing off to work without having eaten properly. Working in a state of tension and pressure all day, smoking, snatching a sandwich and often swilling it down with a pint of beer from the local. Working night shifts, jetting across the world and back, and often working long hours, sometimes seven days a week. Well the personality will have its way, at least for many life-experiences, and time and time again the law of cycles is broken. An animal in its natural state, goes to sleep and eats and rests in very definite cycles and is thus maintaining its equilibrium in respect to the law of rhythm and cycle. Civilised man has managed to transgress the law to a remarkable extent and the state of health of mankind in general is a reflection of this failure to comply to the natural cyclic processes in nature. Modern science tends to encourage man in this, for example 'the pill' which totally interferes with the normal cyclic flow of energies and endocrine functions in woman, breaking an absolutely basic aspect of the law of rhythm inherent in her and in the sex act as well. Medically there may be a few casualties from the pill, the odd thrombotic condition. Statistically rare we are told, but 100% for the woman who dies as a result of the drug upsetting her body. What is not known is just what repercussions might echo down through time into other lives yet to come, nature has an infallible memory and always seeks to bring home its important lessons, and one of these is that the law of cycles cannot be broken without some effect arising, if not now, then certainly later. Another gift to mankind by modern medicine which totally transgresses the law is induced labour in the maternity wards of many hospitals.

This, the prospective young mother is told, will be done for her benefit, and in some cases this is actually the case, or so it would seem. In others, and this is in the majority of cases, it is done in order that the doctor and the staff of the hospital will not be inconvenienced by the erratic arrival of babies according to the decree of nature and the indwelling soul. No doctor wants to be called out in the night or away from his game of golf, when the whole process can be mechanised by an injection to suit the hospital working schedule.

Breaking the law of cycles predisposes man to disease, it creates clashes of energy within his bodies permitting infection to enter. If he would maintain purity of thought he would find that his life out-flowed cyclically in a natural way and there would be nothing in his mental body that could provide a focus for disease patterns to originate around.

DISEASE FACTORS IN THE ASTRAL BODY

Conditions arising in the emotional body of man are one of the most potent sources of disease that the practitioner will have to consider. The activity of this body, when it becomes unduly agitated or tensed has a deleterious effect upon the etheric body which is quick to mirror the disturbances at a subtler level. In his book *The Astral Body* Arthur Powell says:

A developed man has five rates of vibration in his astral body: an ordinary man shows at least nine rates, with a mixture of various shades in addition. Many people have 50 or 100 rates, the whole surface being broken into a multiplicity of little whirlpools and cross-currents, all battling against another in mad confusion. This is the result of unnecessary emotion and worries, the ordinary person of the West being a mass of these, through which much of his strength is frittered away.

An astral body which vibrates fifty ways at once is not only ugly but also a serious annoyance. It may be compared to a physical body suffering from an aggravated form of palsy, with all its muscles jerking simultaneously in different directions. Such astral effects are contagious and affect all sensitive persons who approach, communicating a painful sense of unrest and worry. It is just because millions of people are thus unnecessarily agitated by all sorts of desires and feelings that it is so difficult for a sensitive person to live in a great city or move amongst crowds.

Dr. Edward Bach was one such person who, due to his increasing sensitivity, finally had to leave London and seek the quiet of the countryside. So acute did his quality of sensitivity become that when he placed the petal of a flower upon his tongue, the emotional and mental imbalances that the bloom would cure, manifested themselves in his own being. Although unpleasant and distressing it did enable him to gather together those medicines which later became known as the Bach Remedies.

Powell continues:

> The perpetual astral disturbances may even react through the etheric double and set up nervous diseases.
> The centres of inflammation in the astral body are to it what boils are to the physical body — not only acutely uncomfortable, but also weak spots through which vitality leaks away. They also offer practically no resistance to evil influences and prevent good influences from being of profit. The condition is painfully common: the remedy is to eliminate worry, fear and annoyance.

Alice Bailey in her book *Esoteric Healing* says of the astral body:

> Wrong emotional attitudes and a general unhealthy condition of the astral body must be a potent factor in producing discomfort and disease. . . . Agitation in that body, any violent activity under stress of temper, intense worry or prolonged irritation will pour a stream of astral energy into and through the solar plexus centre, and will galvanise that centre into a condition of intense disturbance. This next effects the stomach, the pancreas, the gall duct and bladder. Few people (and I might well ask who is exempt at this particular time in the world's history) are free from indigestion, from undesirable gastric conditions, or from trouble connected with the gallbladder.

So the prime factors to be considered by any radionic practitioner when he does an analysis, are those which may exist in the astral life of the patient. If hatred, anger, a sense of criticism, fear, superior and inferiority complexes, violent dislikes and a whole host of other emotional forces cloud the clarity of the astral body, then there must be a careful scanning of these points and treatment must be aimed to help the patient drop as many of them as possible from his consciousness. The Bach Remedies are an excellent form of treatment for astral disturbances as we shall see later. On the patient's part the cultivation of an attitude of harmlessness in thought, word and deed will go a long way towards cleansing the astral body and allowing the life forces to flow through unhindered.

When a person's ambitions are bigger than their accomplishments and frustration pervades the astral body for a period of time, a peculiar interaction is set up between the energies of Life and Consciousness that are anchored in the heart and head respectively, and flow along the length of the spine, and the pranic forces entering through the spleen in the region of the solar plexus chakra.

Try to visualise the energies of Life and Consciousness streaming downwards, and those of solar prana coming in through the spleen at right angles to them to form in effect a cross made up of energy streams. These meet in the area of the solar plexus which is the seat of the individual's astral life; if that person has thwarted ambitions, the charge of energy which would flow out normally if such ambitions were realised, begins to back up and accumulate because it is unexpressed. Now because there is such a close link at this point between the heart centre, the blood and the pranic life-forces which must circulate in the blood, the excessive energy charge that is present begins to have an effect upon the blood which under certain conditions may result in malignancy. It is inevitable that a build up of mental, astral, etheric and pranic matter must attract physical matter and so a tumor can be built as a means of expressing the energy of thwarted ambition. This of course is a simplification of the dynamics of some malignancies, there must be any number of other factors and variables which enter into the picture. The cure for many astral conditions including this one is to be found in the cultivation of an attitude of acceptance. Acceptance of what you are, where you are, and the conditions you exist under, not in a negative sense but a dynamic one which hands the reins of your being over to the will of the inner man and allows Life to express Its purpose.

To a clairvoyant the astral body appears as a swirling light form very much the same shape as the dense physical, surrounded by an aura of swirling and flashing colours, looking like the aurora borealis. These colours swiftly change and fluctuate and provide a direct display of the emotional content of the astral body. Theosophists claim that the following colours indicate specific emotional states, which I will list here because they can be used as a guide when analysing this body. In Psionic medicine bacteria and virus are grouped under colour headings in order to speed up and facilitate diagnosis, and Dr. Guyon Richards used the same principle in his work because he found that each micro-organism had a predominant identifying colour or colours. For our purposes, determination of the predominant colours in the astral body will serve as a guide to the patient's emotional nature.

Black:	Hatred and malice.
Red:	Anger.
Scarlet:	Irritability.
Brilliant scarlet:	Noble or righteous indignation.
Lurid red:	Sensuality.
Brown-grey:	Selfishness.
Brown-red:	Avarice.
Greenish-brown with scarlet:	Jealousy.
Grey:	Depression.
Livid grey:	Fear.
Crimson:	Selfish love.
Rose:	Unselfish love.
Rose with lilac:	Spiritual love for humanity.
Orange:	Ambition and pride.
Yellow:	Intellect.
Dull ochre:	Intellect used for selfish purposes.
Clear gamboge:	Intellect used for higher purposes.
Primrose:	Intellect used for spiritual purposes.
Gold:	Intellect applied to philosophy etc.

Green:	Adaptability.
Grey-green:	Deceit and cunning.
Emerald green:	Versatility, ingenuity, resourcefulness used unselfishly.
Pale blue-green:	Adaptability, compassion, deep sympathy.
Apple green:	Strong vitality.
Dark-blue:	Religious feeling.
Light-blue:	Devotion to spiritual ideals.
Violet:	Affection and devotion.
Lilac-blue:	High spiritual aspiration.

Rudolf Steiner points out that in terms of Spiritual Science the relationship between the etheric and astral bodies is bound up in the iron-content of the blood, and that regulation of iron intake affect blood circulation and kidney activity. Cramp-like phenomena are also associated with certain forces in the astral body not functioning properly, so we see that it is possible to begin to understand these subtle aspects of man by observing various objective factors. The writings of Steiner are an invaluable guide which will help any practitioner to bridge the illusory gap between the objective and subjective worlds.

DISEASE FACTORS IN THE ETHERIC BODY

The etheric body is known by a number of names, some refer to it as the vital body or the etheric double, and more recently the term electro-dynamic body has been used, and Russian scientists have called it the bio-plasmic body. Basically it is that body which serves to link the physical organism with the subtler astral and mental forms. It is an absorber of solar energies which it transforms and transmits to all parts of the dense physical by way of its fine energy threads known as the nadis, in modern terminology I suppose one might call it a transducer, for its role is one that is essentially passive, it does not originate action, but simply passes on the impulses from the higher levels to the physical form. Thus it reflects any disease pattern that is to be found in the astral and mental bodies.

To clairvoyant sight it appears as a body of sparkling streams of energy which tend to flow out at right angles to the central nervous system. In sickness this body does not so readily absorb pranic fluids from the sun and as a result the vitality level falls off, and the nadis or energy threads become more attenuated. If this state of affairs is allowed to go on for any length of time the etheric matrix becomes so rarefied that it can no longer support the physical cells and definite organic pathology and disintegration comes about.

In his book *The Vital Body* Rosicrucian Max Heindel writes:

> During health the vital body specializes a superabundance of vital force, which after passing through the dense body, radiates in straight lines in every direction from the periphery thereof, as the radii of a circle do from the centre; but during ill health, when the vital body becomes attenuated, it is not able to draw to itself the same amount of force and in addition the dense physical body is feeding upon it. Then the lines of the vital fluid which pass out from the body are crumpled and bent, showing the lack of force behind them. In health the great force of these radiations carries with it germs and microbes which are inimical to the health of the dense body; but in sickness, when the vital force is weak, these emanations do not so readily eliminate disease germs. Therefore the danger of contracting disease is much greater when the vital forces are low than when one is in robust health.

I have dealt with the dynamics of pranic reception and distribution in *Radionics and the Subtle Anatomy of Man* so there is no need for me to go into any more details here. The question that arises at this point is, if the etheric body is a reflector of states of imbalance in other bodies, does disease itself originate in the etheric body independently? The answer to this is quite simply, yes! There are a number of reasons why, and it is important for any practitioner to understand them, for they are factors that will be present in most cases that are radionically analysed.

The first thing to realise is that our etheric and dense physical bodies are drawn from the etheric and physical substance of the planet. This material, according to esoteric tradition, is very old in origin and because of this it is contaminated to a very high degree. For countless aeons the diseased bodies of men and animals have been placed under the soil, and this has brought about a very profound yet subtle pollution of the matter which we attract to build our vehicles of manifestation. Esoteric tradition goes further and states that all disease can be placed under three categories, those of syphilis, tuberculosis and cancer, and that these are all inherent in the etheric and physical substance of our planet. So potentially all are liable to pick up these predisposing patterns in their etheric and physical bodies, and the life-style will serve either to trigger them into activity or allow them to remain dormant. Here alone is surely an indication of the value of pure living habits which will serve to keep the etheric body in a radiant state.

In her book *Esoteric Healing* Alice Bailey writes:

> It should be borne in mind that the physical bodies in which humanity now dwells are constructed of very ancient matter and that the substance employed is tainted or conditioned by the history of the past. To this concept must be added two others: First, that incoming souls draw to themselves the type of material with which they must construct their outer sheaths, and that this will be responsive to some aspect of their subtler natures. . . . Secondly, each physical body carries within itself the seeds of inevitable retribution, if its functions are misused.

Samuel Hahnemann the founder of homoeopathy recognised that man carries the seeds of disease within, and he called these predisposing patterns, miasms. These are known as Psora, Pseudo-Psora, Syphilis and Sycosis. Hahnemann called Psora "The Mother of all diseases," without which no other disease can manifest. Of it, he said: "Psora it is, that oldest, most universal, most pernicious and yet least known chronic miasmatic disease, which has been deforming and torturing the nations for thousands of years." He was also very aware that these dyscrasias were not physical but subtle in origin and related to the vital force. Of this he wrote:

> When a person falls ill, it is only this spiritual, self-acting (automatic) vital force, everywhere present in his organism, that is primarily deranged by the dynamic influence upon it of a morbific agent inimical to life; it is only the vital force, deranged to such an abnormal state, that can furnish the organism with its disagreeable sensations, and incline it to the irregular processes which we call disease.

Miasms and taints may be inherited or acquired, and their presence always undermines the health of the individual to a greater or lesser extent, not only from a physical point of view but also on emotional and mental levels as well. Every childhood disease we contract may leave in its wake toxins which have a very deleterious effect upon health, measles being a particularly unpleasant disease which has strong effects later in life*. Orthodox medicine naturally says that there is no scientific proof of this claim made by radiesthetists and radionic practitioners, but in America doctors have finally traced the mysterious deaths of college students just turned 20 years of age (some 200 each year), to what they term a 'smouldering measles virus' which has lain dormant since they had the disease in earlier years, or from the time they received a vaccination of the attenuated virus. These deaths are extreme cases involving apparently healthy young adults in the main, people simply suffering poor health all their lives from various viral or bacterial toxins, which are disturbing the etheric body and devitalising it, ultimately to the point where organic problems may make their appearance.

At the time of writing there is a controversy raging in the press about the damage done to children by vaccinations. Infants are irreperably damaged by the effects of some vaccinations and reduced to the status of a cabbage for the rest of their lives. The particular vaccine that has been attacked is the one given for whooping cough, but if the truth be known all vaccinations have the effect of diminishing the vital force within the etheric body. Proponents for vaccination point out, and quite rightly, that only a small minority of children are badly affected, but this is the same old story as with the pill and thrombosis, if its you or your child, then the figure is 100%. To see an otherwise healthy infant paralysed or destroyed by a vaccination because it happens to be current medical practice, is a pathetic spectacle. Brain damage is never a pretty sight, and to know that a life has been cut off as the result of an act of the State which encourages parents, and in many cases literally frightens them into having

*The Contribution of Psionic Medicine to Hahnemann's Miasmic Theory by Aubrey T. Westlake, B.A., M.B., B.Chir.(Cantab). M.R.C.S., L.C.R.P. from Journal of The Psionic Medical Society, Winter 1974.

their children vaccinated, makes one wonder. Surely even one million pounds spent on investigating the use of homoeopathic nosodes for the childhood diseases would be money well deployed. They are as effective as vaccinations, at least from my own very limited experience, they would appear to be so, and there are no side effects whatsoever. Naturally orthodoxy does not want to know about this because it is not scientific.

Radionic and radiesthetic techniques are ideally suited to trace the presence of any miasms or toxins in the system. Dr. George Laurence spent years perfecting Psionic Medicine*, through which he helped many people to recover their health. All cases analysed showed that miasmic or toxic patterns were present that disturbed the function of the etheric formative forces of the body and ultimately the protein of the cell. Laurence was able to determine not only the imbalances but also the homoeopathic remedies that would erradicate the miasms or bacterial and viral toxins. From personal experience I know how effective this form of treatment is, and that the same results can also be obtained by radionic means as well. It would be interesting to see just how much help could be given to children who show clear signs of brain damage due to vaccination. Asthma and eczema have been traced to vaccinations and cured by Psionic Medicine. The other important point too is that inherited disease patterns can be detected and eliminated in children so that they are not passed on to future generations.

The integrity of the etheric body is maintained and enhanced by a natural diet, organically grown wholefoods, fresh air, sunshine, honey as a sweetner, exercise, a relaxed attitude, the judicious use of water both internally and externally and a regulated rhythm of breathing. Emotional and mental turmoil will debilitate the vital body, drugs give the nadis an appearance rather like the strings of a tennis racquet that are slack, and it should ever be kept in mind that the etheric body responds rapidly to thought. The yearly warnings by medical 'experts' through the media of television and radio, that polio or flu

*Psionic Medicine by J.H. Reyner BSC, D.I.C., F.I.E.E. in collaboration with George Laurence M.R.C.S., L.R.C.P., F.R.C.S. (Edin) and Carl Upton L.D.S. (Birm). Published by Routledge & Keegan Paul, London.

epidemics are on their way, is a sure fire method for setting up a suitable state of receptivity to these diseases in the populace. Spurred on by fear of the disease many get their flu shots and wind up with the infection anyhow; others report that they have never felt well since they had the injection, which is only natural when one considers that a poisonous substance has been introduced into the body.

The growing awareness of the public to the dangers inherent in the use of vaccines and to the side effects of prescribed drugs, is indicative of changes that are in the offing. The whole new awareness that people have with regards to vitamins, natural unprocessed foods and the practice of yoga is indicative of the approaching revelation of the etheric body. When this comes about, medicine itself will alter radically, becoming less physical in its approach to healing.

THE CHAKRAS AND DISEASE

A proper understanding of the seven major spinal chakras and their functions is essential to the radionic practitioner, for it is the chakras that hold the body together in one coherent, vitalised whole. These centres are focal points through which the soul works to express its life and quality on the lower planes of consciousness. Through them the life energies pour, maintaining the action of the endocrine glands and the integrity of certain areas of the body. The health of any individual is totally dependent upon their correct functioning. As long as the reception, assimilation and distribution of these energies takes place in a balanced way, then health manifests itself quite naturally. A number of problems can arise in respect of the functioning of the chakras which will create disease and it is these factors that I want to deal with now, bearing in mind that in the proper action of the centre lies one of the major keys to health.

An imbalance in the function of a chakra can occur for a number of reasons, each of which can be modified for the better, or cleared up through radionic treatment.

1.   Attitudes and activities predominating in this, or past lives, may set up a state of overactivity in any one, or several chakras. For the same reason some may be underactive.

Thus it is important to know in any diagnosis the state of each chakra, which will fall into one of three categories: OVERACTIVE – UNDERACTIVE – NORMALLY ACTIVE. To determine these states of activity is absolutely basic to any diagnosis of the centres and the subtle anatomy in general.

2. Damage can occur to the peculiarly sensitive substance that goes into the makeup of a chakra. This can arise due to physical trauma, sudden or sustained emotional stress or shock. For example an otherwise healthy male patient in his mid-forties, engaged in manual labour, developed acute attacks of asthma from the day he found a relative dead. The shock had radically disturbed the function of his throat chakra.

3. As a result of the above factors chakras may become blocked and their capacity to receive and distribute energy is impaired. If the blockage occurs at the entrance to the centre then the inflowing energy will not find access. Instead of flowing on out into expression it backs up like water in a stream that has been dammed, and sets up a focus of irritation at its point of origin which may have been on astral or mental levels. Blockages can also occur at the point where energy exits from the chakra and touches upon the endocrine gland, in these cases the energy builds up at that point until it reaches an intensity which will enable it to push past the blockage. This results in erratic function of the endocrine gland associated with the chakra in question. Chakras then can be BLOCKED AT ENTRANCE or BLOCKED AT EXIT, either condition will create imbalances in energy flow and ultimately pathological states of a mental, emotional or physical nature.

Much ill health also arises during the process of energy transference from the chakras below the diaphragm to those above. This normally takes place very slowly in the initial stages but speeds up as the individual disciplines his life in order to deliberately move more quickly forward on the Path. The whole process of energy transference is very complex and by no means a straightforward cut and dried issue, however it can be broadly outlined in such a way that the information is of practical use.

As I have mentioned in *Radionics and the Subtle Anatomy of Man* the chakras below the diaphragm are concerned with the more mundane factors in life, procreation and the digestive processes among them. The energies of the base chakra are transferred to the crown, those of the sacral to the throat and those of solar plexus to the heart. Diagramatically we have the following outline.

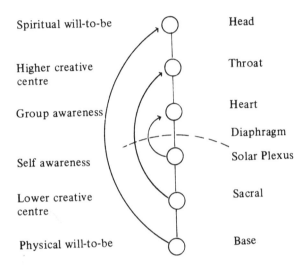

In this instance the two head chakras are shown under one heading, simply because the outline is a broad and general one. At one point in the multiplicity of energy transfers all the qualities of energies found in the base, sacral, solar plexus, heart and throat are focussed in the brow chakra prior to their 'submission' to those of the crown. The microcosmic crisis occurs when the personality or low-self surrenders to the soul, and the New Man emerges into greater and completely unselfish service to humanity.

Every case that presents itself for radionic analysis will involve to a greater or lesser degree, problems arising from energy transference. The centres below the diaphragm will in many instances be very active and when this energy beging to make an impact on the higher counterpart, which obviously is not going to be so active, then a great deal of friction occurs creating all manner of physical and psychological problems. Always remember ENERGY TRANSFERENCE IS CONSCIOUSNESS TRANS-FERENCE and when the focus of consciousness in any energy system alters there are inevitable problems. Keep in mind too that these problems are not going to readily give way to radionic therapy, because they are part and parcel of the evolution of the individual and cannot be brushed aside at the flick of a tuning dial. However once the practitioner has understood what is going on then he or she is in a better position to help. Now in helping a patient along such lines I am not suggesting that they be told of all the blockages and energy transferences that are going on in their systems, this is a sure way to add to their troubles. Once you tell a patient that he has trouble with a certain chakra, you are immediately focussing his attention upon the nature of the problem and where it lies. This will in the long run only exacerbate the trouble. Often patients want to know what is wrong, and it may be all right to tell them of the miasms or toxins that are undermining their health, but the minute you start dealing with problems relative to their chakras you are only going to inject energy into thoughtforms that are pathological in nature and thus slow down any progress the patient might make. The emphasis must be upon a return to health, the underlying causes should be relegated to the filing cabinet and not impressed upon the substance of the patient's subtle bodies, he will have enough to deal with without fuel being added to the fire.

From first hand experience I can give an example of energy transference in an individual who knew in full consciousness that he was a disciple in a certain ashram on the inner planes. Outwardly he was an ordinary retired businessman and that was his image to 99% of the people who knew him. My association with him over the years led me to an understanding of his health problem which was emphysema. In a previous life he had through a tremendous effort on his part, succeeded in bringing about a major transfer of energy from his sacral chakra to the throat. In this life he was experiencing the repercussions of this shift in consciousness, which greatly overloaded the throat chakra and gave rise to the disease he suffered from. Coinciding with this problem was the fact that he was preparing to move from one ashram to begin serving in another wherein the will aspect dominated. His disease which incapacitated him to the point where he thought at times he would die on the spot from lack of air, made him call upon the quality of spiritual will in order to keep going and rise above his disability. In this way he was able to use the crisis which filled most of his life, to develop certain qualities that would extend his capacity to help others, particularly in future incarnations.

I am not suggesting that by giving this example, all emphysema patients are in the same position as this individual, far from it, but it does show what happens when a major transfer takes place and how a spiritually evolved person makes constructive use of the disability. A person of this calibre takes advantage of every opportunity to learn and does not focus his or her attention on the problem but on the reality and reasons that lie beyond it. I believe that supportive treatment through radionics can be of use in such cases, but the patient should not be informed of the findings made by the practitioner. In this instance the individual knew what was wrong and how to deal with it, others may not be so capable.

This is not the place to go into specific diseases associated with the different chakras, I have covered this in my other books to a limited degree and the reader can find a lot of information along these lines in various esoteric books. What I would stress however is that the chart showing the chakras, their glands and the areas governed by the chakras, is an excellent and simple guide. For example, if there is gall-bladder trouble then you will know immediately that the solar plexus chakra is probably overactive, which is so often the case. If eye problems occur then the brow chakra must in some way or other be in a state of imbalance. ALWAYS LOOK TO THE CHAKRA NEAREST TO THE AREA WHERE PATHOLOGY MANIFESTS is a good rule of thumb to follow, half the time in analysing a health problem in the subtle anatomy you don't need clairvoyance or intuition but just plain common sense.

THREE PRIMARY STATES OF IMBALANCE

Broadly speaking it is possible to classify most of the problems arising in the subtle anatomy under three headings, which are as follows.

1.   CONGESTION which arises due to a lack of free flow of the energies and forces in the various bodies. Congestion of the etheric body can arise where energies flow in from the astral vehicle or plane, it can also occur between the astral and etheric bodies or between the etheric and the physical. Congestion of any type will give rise to symptoms on the physical plane.

2.   UN-COORDINATION can occur between any two vehicles creating a weakness which manifests as poor health. If the dense physical and etheric bodies are not well integrated then debilitation and devitalisation take place. Impotence is a reflection of this problem in the area of the sacral chakra. In the throat centre which is the polar opposite to the sacral, a similar condition would give rise to laryngitis. If the general coordination of vehicles is poor, the soul may have a loose grip upon them, in such cases possession or obsession can come about.

3.   OVERSTIMULATION arises when there is too much energy being drawn in through a particular chakra or chakras, this agitates the substance of the bodies involved and in so doing brings about a variety of pathological conditions. Fevers for example are an expression of an over active focal point of energy that is trying to disperse and flow outward into physical expression. The accompanying friction naturally causes a rise in temperature.

All cases must be checked for these factors, because like blockages and states of activity they are basic fundamental problems which lie behind symptom patterns that patients present.

This concludes a basic outline of those factors that must be taken into consideration when dealing with the analysis of conditions that lie in the subtle bodies of man. These are the causative factors, or at least some of them, which we would place under the heading of physical and psychological problems.

There are other factors that come into the causes of disease such as individual, group, national, racial and planetary karma which I personally feel lie beyond our jurisdiction, at least they do at this point in time. It is enough I think, to deal with what we can in some measure understand, to become involved in trying to deal with causes that lie completely beyond our comprehension is to court trouble.

Competent handling of the processes and procedures of diagnosis and treatment as outlined in this book will enable the practitioner to bring a good measure of healing to the patients that come for help, in a simple yet effective manner. This in itself has a great deal to commend it, especially when you realise that causative factors are being dealt with, not just symptom patterns, and that the removal of inherited and acquired miasms and toxins clear the 'soil' of the body, so that they are not handed on to future generations.

These then are some of the basic concepts that the practitioner will need. To understand them more fully it will be necessary for the reader to delve into and study the writings of Rudolf Steiner that are relative to medicine, those of Alice Bailey and indeed of others who have covered the subject of healing in depth. Sort through the information you find, sift out that which you cannot make practical use of, and employ the fundamentals at all times. It is a vast subject and more than a life times study, but each day is a day of opportunity and preparation for future greater usefulness and effectiveness.

SECTION FOUR

Therapeutic Considerations

The keynote to good health, esoterically speaking, is sharing or distribution, just as it is the keynote to the general well-being of humanity. The economic ills of mankind closely correspond to disease in the individual. There is a lack of free flow of the necessities of life to the points of distribution; these points of distribution are idle; the direction of the distribution is faulty, and only through a sane and world-wide grasp of the New Age principle of sharing will human ills be cured; only by the right distribution of energy will the ills of the physical body of individual man also be cured.

Alice A. Bailey

One develops spiritual sight, looks into the spiritual world, arrives at a conception of man, of the being of man in health and disease, and then it is possible to found a kind of spiritual medicine.

Rudolf Steiner

CHAPTER NINE

Avenues of Approach

Who ever saw one physician approve of another's prescription, without taking something away, or adding something to it?

Montaigne

The radionic practitioner is faced with a considerable range of choice when it comes to treatment. For his part he may use rates or ratios which he projects by means of a radionic instrument, or he may apply the patterns of gems, colours, flower remedies, vitamins, tissue salts or homoeopathic medicines. On the other hand, if they are indicated, he will recommend that the patient seek a specialist in acupuncture, diet, manipulation or an allopathic doctor. Thus no avenue of approach is barred in the effort to restore health to the patient.

One soon learns in radionics that although there might be a few specific treatments for particular conditions, in general the practitioner has to allow the disease pattern to select its own form of therapy, which is of course done through the approach of question and answer and the Analyser, setting certain remedies against the causative factor in order to arrive at a measurement which indicates balance. Inevitably when dealing with subjective factors some unusual remedies are at times indicated, but more often than not, a quick look at the 'findings' for that remedy in Boericke's *Materia Medica* will reveal many of the symptoms exhibited by the patient under consideration, thus confirming the suitability of the radiesthetically chosen remedy.

Some practitioners use broadcast or projections of ratios or various remedies exclusively, others employ a combination of projected treatment and the use of oral medicines, it is simply a matter of preference and choice. As the concept of projecting a treatment to patients at a distance by means of instrumentation is unique to radionics, perhaps it is best to clarify what that involves, in other words to define radionic treatment. Our definition is that A RADIONIC TREATMENT IS THE PRO-JECTION OF A SET OF CODED INSTRUCTIONS, DESIGNED TO BE TAKEN UP, AND ACTED UPON BY THE VARIOUS ENERGY FIELDS OF THE PATIENT IN A WAY THAT WILL ENABLE A STATE OF HARMONY AND HEALTH TO MANI-FEST IN THE PHYSICAL BODY.

The archetypal blueprint of the body is perfect; deviation from that blueprint brings about dis-ease. The treatment, particularly if it is an organ ratio, is a way of presenting a model to the imbalance, to the intelligence pervading the cells lacking harmony, and reminding them of the way they should function, and of their inherent perfect morphology. Projections of flower remedies, tissue salts or colour are just another way of doing the same thing, pulsing the treatment serves to drive home the message and bring it clearly to the attention of the substance of the bodies.

I want to consider now, some of the forms of treatment that are used in radionics, and to put down material from various sources that should prove useful to practitioners in the daily round of their work.

COLOUR – THE UNIVERSAL REMEDY

Colour as a form of treatment in radionics has always been my own particular favourite approach, and over the years it has proved to be effective in a wide variety of cases. Somehow it seems so closely associated with the subtle bodies and their radiant shifting colours. In his book *Spiritual Science and Medicine* Rudolf Steiner says:

> The delicacy and sensitiveness of our bodily organisation become evident also by objective and systematic study of light and colour treatment for disease. This use of light and colour should be more considered in the future than it has in the past.

And:

> In my opinion much importance should be attached to these methods in a not distant future. Colour therapy, not only light-treatment, will soon play a great part.

One of the most famous colour therapists of all time was a Dr. Edwin Babbitt who lived in America in the late 1800's. His book, *The Principles of Light and Colour* made him world famous when it first appeared in 1878. Babbitt was an odd combination of scientist, artist, physician and mystic and it is clear from his writings that he had direct access to knowledge that was only available to those who could penetrate the inner worlds in full consciousness. In his treatment he used lamps with special colour lenses to great effect, he also irradiated sac lac tablets and liquids with colour in order to make remedies that were taken orally by his patients.

The following lists of diseases and the colours he used are drawn from his book, and should serve as a guideline to radionic practitioners, especially in emergency treatments and to compliment whatever other form of therapy, radionic or otherwise, that has been decided upon in various cases under the practitioner's care.

Blue (+ additional colours)

Apoplexy	Headaches
Brain diseases	Hepatitis
Bronchitis (+ White)	Hot inflammation
Chronic rheumatism (+ Yellow & White)	
	Hysteria
Cystitis (+ Yellow)	Inflammation of ovaries
Catarrh (+ White)	Inflammatory rheumatism
Diarrhoea	Menorrhagia

Diphtheria (+ Yellow &
  White)
Erysiphelas
Facial neuralgia
Fevers: Typhoid
           Yellow (+ White)
           Bilious
           Intermittent
Gout
Haemorrhage of lungs

Nervous excitability
Palpitations of heart
Pustules, watery pimples
Pertussis (+ White)
Pneumonia (+ White)
Pleurisy (+ White)
Sciatica (+ White)
Spinal problems
Small Pox
Scabies

Red (+ additional colours)
Goitres

Arousing circulation of arterial
  blood

Dormant tumours
Amenorrhea (+ Yellow)

Yellow (+ additional colours)
Arousing activity of nervous system
Aphonia (+ White)
Constipation
Diabetes (+ White)
Fatty degeneration of heart (+ White)
Goitres
Paralysis (+ White)
Tuberculosis (+ White)
Pertussis (+ White)

Purple
Stimulate circulation of venous blood
Worms

Yellow-Orange
Anaemia

Hypo-function of liver, kidneys
  lower spine
Hard chronic tumors
Idiocy

Bronchitis
Constipation

Depression   Ulceration of lungs
Dropsy
Exhaustion

Another great colour therapist was Dr. C.E. Iredell, a cancer specialist for 23 years, who was surgeon-emeritus of the actino-theraputic department at Guy's Hospital in London during the 1920's. Despite the fact that most of the patients he treated with colour had already undergone orthodox treatment, and in many cases were burned as a result, he was able to report excellent results, and in some cases cures. His first experiments he recorded in the following words.

> The first experiment with colour was made by placing a piece of violet glass against a malignant swelling in a patient's neck and holding an ordinary electric glow lamp by it for an hour. The patient experienced definite soothing effects, and the experiment was therefore repeated in other cases. Tests were also carried out with other colours, especially green and blue. Each colour appeared to have a definite individual effect clearly distinguishable to a sensitive patient, though no appreciable diminution in the size of the swelling treated was observed at this stage. Sometimes however, the surrounding inflammation was reduced, and in almost every case was attended by relief of pain and improvement in general condition. It was of interest to note that the more intense the colours used the more effective they seemed to be.

Iredell found that some patients could relate in detail the sensations they perceived when colour was used upon them, and frequently with practice could tell one colour from another in this manner.

> Sometimes a patient was found who, in addition to feeling relief of pain, was conscious of a definite sensation produced by Colour on the body as a whole which was stimulating and invigorating. Less frequently a patient was found who was able to distinguish in the sensation above referred to the different effects of the various colours, each colour having distinct characteristics of its own.
>
> It may be of interest here to give some rough idea of the effects of the colours used as described by some of the patients who were sufficiently sensitive to feel them. The colour most generally used was a bright green. The sensation it produced was generally described as cool and pleasant, but not very smooth. It was soothing when the patient was restless. It was also the colour with which it was found advisable to begin and end all treatments, as the effects of the other

colours were intensified if an application of green was given after
they had been used.

A deep royal blue generally followed the use of green. The
sensation produced by this shade was cooler and smoother than that
of green, but it was liable to produce depression if given for more
than a short time. Yellow, which was sometimes employed after
blue, seemed, in the earlier cases, to do harm, as it was too "strong".
This was probably due to the fact that the strength in which it was
given was too great, the patients stating that it made the pain worse.
It was found later, however, that if the other colours were used first,
and especially blue, the action of which was stabilising and restful
when only a short application was given, yellow produced very
definite beneficial results which were different from those obtained
by any other colour. The shade of yellow used was a deep amber,
and it produced a feeling of warmth which was distinguishable from
that produced by diathermy and, while it was a tonic in action, it had,
at the same time, a soothing effect.

The sensation produced by violet, which was used after yellow,
was far smoother and finer than that produced by green, which it
closely resembled in other respects. The use of violet was not nearly
so effective unless it was used in conjunction with, and after, all the
other colours, when, from a clinical point of view, its effects were
particularly striking.

The two remaining colours, red and orange, were little used,
although red seemed to be useful in treating anaemic patients and
was also valuable in preventing sickness. Orange acted as a general
stimulant and was effective when indigestion was present. Its effect
was coarser than that of yellow.

It will be noticed that the arrangement of the colours was not that
of those in the visible spectrum, which are red, orange, yellow, green,
blue, indigo, and violet. There is no apparent reason for the alteration
in the place of yellow when the position of the other colours corres-
ponds to the arrangement of the spectrum.

It was not expected from the results obtained, even when the
drawbacks of the apparatus had been corrected, that Colour treatment alone would be a cure for malignant disease. In this respect it
corresponded closely to the other agents used for cancer which
invariably do good at first and, just as certainly, tend with time to
lose their beneficial effect. In other words, the cancer gets used to
any form of treatment, and even, in some cases, seems to be stimulated
by it. Yet the results obtained by Colour were so encouraging that it
was thought worth while pursuing the investigation to try to discover
some means, which, when used conjointly, would overcome the
difficulties encountered.

Eventually from all his experimental work, Iredell developed
an instrument for applying colour to his patients, he called this

the Focal Machine which consisted of three discs with triangular shapes cut from them, in these the colour transparencies were placed. Behind them were powerful light sources and motors to drive the discs; as these spun the colour falling upon the patient's body was subjected to a rhythm, in other words it was pulsed. So important was this rhythm that Iredell found that if he synchronised it with the pulse-rate and had the patient regulate his respiration rate, the treatment was more effective. I want to include here a lengthy extract from *Colour and Cancer* because I feel that it contains material that is relative to the pulsing of radionic treatments, and that what Iredell has to say might serve to stimulate individuals in the various healing arts to apply his concepts to their own particular work.

The idea of introducing rhythm into medicine is not new, and heart disease in particular is an instance of its importance. Cardiac irregularity is looked on as a symptom that needs treatment, and a marked improvement in the patient's general condition is often seen as the heartbeat returns to normal. Other instances of the importance of rhythm could be enumerated. From the point of view of physics it is a well-known fact that every body has a vibration rate of its own, and even if it is made up of different substances which vibrate at different rates, nevertheless that body as a whole will have a definite rate depending on the physical characteristics of its component parts. A simple instance of this is a jelly. It is a matter of common knowledge that a jelly when shaken moves rhythmically and, as a matter of fact, the vibration rate is always the same for the same jelly. If a rubber tube is coiled in it and connected with a pump and the tube is filled with water, each time the pump is squeezed movement is seen in the jelly. If this is noticed carefully it will be observed that one movement of the pump produces not a single movement but a series of diminishing vibrations or waves. If the ends of the pump are connected with the ends of a rubber tube so that a continuous circulation is possible, we have a closed system corresponding to the vascular system of the human body. If the pump is squeezed seventy or eighty times a minute we have a resemblance to the heartbeat, and between each beat a series of lesser vibrations. In cases of advanced aortic disease and aortic aneurism one can sometimes observe a shake of the head with each heartbeat and, if this is watched carefully, a succession of vibrations beginning with each beat may occasionally be seen. The same series of movements also occurs in the foot of the normal subject when one leg is crossed over the other. Presumably, therefore, while the bones, muscles, etc., have different rates of vibration, the body as a whole has a certain rate of vibration which is a multiple of the pulse-rate. The pulse in the femoral artery is one-sixth of a second after the contraction of the left ventricle and, taking the pulse-rate as eighty, the figure 480 (obtained by multiplying 80 by 6) was taken as an hypothesis for future work in this connection. It is not claimed that these suggestions are of any importance scientifically, but they formed a basis on which a working figure was obtained. The importance of this figure will be seen later.

To carry out experiments a large cardboard disc two feet in diameter was obtained, and a hole four inches square was cut in it near the circumference. The disc was mounted at its centre on the spindle of a small electric motor. The combination was arranged so that an electric light behind a hole in the disc fell on the swelling to be treated. In front of the light was placed the coloured glass. The disc was revolved at different rates, and it was found that when the rate was such that the light fell synchronously with the pulse, a more marked beneficial effect was produced than when the light fell on the swelling continuously. This was afterwards confirmed in many other cases.

The success of this investigation suggested that, if the rhythm of respiration could be brought into play, the results would be even better. It should be borne in mind that between the rhythms of the pulse and respiration there is this marked difference — that the former cannot be regulated voluntarily, while the latter is under the control of the will. The pulse-rate is about seventy or eighty, while the respiration is twenty a minute. If the pulse-rate is assumed to be eighty, the respiration can be kept at twenty or, in other words, one complete breath, consisting of an inspiration and an expiration, can be made to four heartbeats.

Various modifications were made in the cardboard disc with the idea of bringing these considerations into Colour treatment, and experiments, such as using slots of different sizes and the substitution of two or three cardboard discs for the one disc originally employed, were tried. It was found that the introduction of means to establish a synchronisation with the respiration-rate was an advantage, while an optimum-rate, much faster than the pulse-rate, but above or below which results seemed to be less satisfactory, could be discovered for each patient. This rate, which could easily be adjusted and correctly regulated, corresponded roughly to 480 a minute, and seemed therefore to confirm the hypothetical figure which to reference has already been made.

As Iredell's experiments continued his Focal Machine became more complicated. Patients were placed in light-proof circular enclosures, magnetic and radio waves were introduced along with the colour and it was found that if the colour was first passed down a rotating funnel with a spiral inside, that the effect was magnified many times. The famous radiesthetist Enel who specialised in the treatment of cancer also employed energies given off from spirals, perhaps the rotary movement has some direct link with the action of the chakras and serves to balance their function. Many of Iredell's patients when under treatment used to begin touching their bodies to see if they were wet. It seems that the release and stimulated flow of energy through their bodies gave the sensation that water was running over them. To my mind the colour must have released the flow of life-force or prana which they had blocked off for many years, and like Wilhelm Reich's patients they began to experience what he called 'orgonotic streamings', the free and outward flow of the universal life-force.

Although Iredell worked mostly with cancer patients he also from time to time treated other diseases with colour, such as glaucoma, polio, neuritis, iritis and nasal catarrh. He reports that practically all cases of rheumatism responded well to treatments with the colours rose and blue.

While Iredell had worked quietly at his researches, a colour therapist came to prominence in America in the 1930's who was a trifle more flamboyant and not adverse to publicity. His name was Dinshah P. Ghadiali who boasted an M.S-C after his name, meaning Master of Spectro-Chrome Metry and not to be confused with Master of Science. This was followed by another eleven (listed) honorary degrees ranging from M.D., Ph.D., through D.C., to D.Opt., the rest, obviously too many to mention came under the heading of Etc. He claimed to be a metaphysician and psychologist, and was a member or leading light of numerous organisations ranging all the way from Fellow and Ex-Vice-President, Allied Medical Associations of America to Member of The Independent Order of Rechabites, whoever or whatever they might have been. He was a Good Templar, an anti-vivisectionist, an anti-vaccinationist and a student of Theosophy. His brochures show him sitting in his study, and under his photograph the words Dinshah — Humble Servant Of Suffering Humanity. His platform as adopted by him in 1891 is revealed by the words: (All capitals)

The Boundless Oscillatory Ocean Of Thought Is Essentially Universal And All-Pervading. It Is The Individualized Monopoly Of NO Person And Is The Common Heritage Of Humanity's Evolution; Thus, What A Development Of Unrevealed Ages Has Been Given Unto Me In The Form Of Knowledge In My Present Incarnation Is No Distinctive Acquisition Of Mine For My Sole Use, Benefit Or Elevation, But Is All For Thee And Is Thine Without Condition, Without Obligation, Without Expectation. I Fear No One; Only God Above And Conscience Below And From Them I Have Nothing To Fear.

He challenged the world to dispute the claims he made for his method of colour therapy, and no doubt he would have been able to substantiate most of them. Unfortunately a long string of letters after one's name, loud claims for therapeutic success and a most persistent habit of harangueing the Establishment, attracts the authorities like flies. Somewhere along the line Dinshah collected one 'honorary degree' too many, or made an overly extravagant claim, or struck a sore spot in the body of the Establishment and the next he knew was that men with sledge hammers had a court order to smash all of his colour therapy equipment, and Dinshah was put out of business. Had he been a little more circumspect he may have survived to help more people regain their health, because despite his attitudes Dinshah Ghadiali had a lot to offer and there is clear evidence from his writings that he had developed, like Edwin Babbitt, a very effective approach to colour healing. For purposes of use in a radionic practice there are two lists from his writings which I feel will be helpful. The first deals with the use of each colour in respect to body systems and disease conditions, the other with the colour waves of chemical elements.

Under the heading 'Spectro-Chrome Tonation System . . . The Culmination of Dinshah's Laborious Researchs' the following information is given.

GREEN:
Pituitary stimulant
Disinfectant
Purificatory
Antiseptic
Germicide

LEMON:
Cerebral stimulant
Thymus activator
Antacid
Chronic alterative
Antiscorbutic

Green.

Bactericide

Detergent

Muscle and tissue builder

Lemon

Laxative

Expectorant

Bone builder

YELLOW:

Motor stimulant

Ailmentary tract energizer

Lymphatic activator

Splenic depressant

Digestant

Cathartic

Cholegogue

Anthelmintic

Nerve builder

ORANGE:

Respiratory stimulant

Parathyroid depressant

Thyroid energizer

Antispasmodic

Galactagogue

Antirachitic

Emetic

Carminative

Stomachic

Aromatic

Lung builder

RED:

Sensory stimulant

Liver energizer

Irritant

Vesicant

Pustulant

Rubefacient

Caustic

Haemoglobin builder

SCARLET:

Arterial stimulant

Renal energizer

Genital excitant

Aphrodisiac

Emmenagogue

Vasoconstrictor

Ecbolic

MAGENTA:

Superarenal stimulant

Cardiac energizer

Diuretic

Emotional equilibrator

Auric builder

PURPLE:

Venous stimulant

Renal depressant

Anti malarial

Vasodilator

Anaphrodisiac

Narcotic

Hypnotic

Antipyretic

Analgesic

VIOLET:
Splenic stimulant
Cardiac depressant
Lymphatic depressant
Motor depressant
Leucocyte builder

INDIGO:
Parathyroid stimulant
Thyroid depressant
Respiratory depressant
Astringent
Sedative
Pain reliever
Hemostatic
Inspissator
Phagocyte builder

BLUE:
Antipruritic
Diaphoretic
Febrifuge
Counter-irritant
Anodyne
Demulcent
Vitality builder

TURQUOISE:
Cerebral depressant
Acute alterative
Acid
Tonic
Skin builder

As all radionic treatment is determined on the specific need for a specific case, these uses for the various colours should simply serve as a guideline, or they may be used as I have said before as an adjunct to other treatment or in an emergency. If a patient is in acute pain, then indigo can be used as a general treatment while other remedies are being checked out. At times a practitioner may be faced with an emergency in the family, when the mind may not be calm enough to quickly and accurately determine the treatment needed, so reference to the list above may prove useful as an interim way of picking out a treatment.

Dinshah's correlation of the various elements with colours may also prove useful in a similar way. Quite frequently patients are found to be lacking in certain elements, if these are to be projected or broadcast to the patient then it will help if the element needed is given alongside a treatment with the related colour, thus supplementing and augmenting its healing capacity.

GREEN:
Barium
Chlorine
Kashmirium
Nitrogen
Radium
Tellurium
Thallium

LEMON:
Cerium
Germanium
Gold
Iodine
Iron
Lanthanum
Neodymium
Phosphorus
Praseodymium
Samarium
Scandium
Silver
Sulphur
Thorium
Titanium
Uranium
Vanadium
Yttrium
Zirconium

YELLOW:
Carbon
Glucinum
Iridium
Magnesium
Molybdenum
Osmium
Palladium
Platinum
Rhodium
Ruthenium
Sodium
Tin
Tungsten

ORANGE:
Aluminium
Antimony
Arsenic
Boron
Calcium
Copper
Helium
Selenium
Silicon
Xenon

RED:
Cadmium
Hydrogen
Krypton
Neon

SCARLET:
Argon
Dysprosium
Erbium
Holmium
Lutecium
Manganese
Thulium
Ytterbium

MAGENTA:
Irenium
Lithium
Potassium
Rubidium
Strontium

PURPLE:
Bromine
Europium
Gadolinium
Terbium

VIOLET:
Actinium
Cobalt
Gallium
Niton

INDIGO:	*BLUE:*	*TURQUOISE:*
Bismuth	Caesium	Chromium
Ionium	Indium	Columbium
Lead	Oxygen	Fluorine
Polonium		Mercury
		Nickel
		Tantalum
		Zinc

Most colour therapists use a fairly narrow range of colours, in radionics this range is extended considerably, and if colour treatments are applied by means of the magneto-geometric potency simulator, the practitioner has 300 shades of colour in the form of ratio cards to select his treatment from, which must constitute a distinct advantage over other approaches.

In *Letters on Occult Meditation* Alice Bailey deals at some length with the uses of colour in meditation and healing. She points out that the seven colours of the spectrum represent the seven great streams of energy that vitalise our solar system known as the Seven Rays. The Bible calls them The Seven Spirits before the Throne of God, and the Christian mystic Jacob Boehme refers to them as The Fountain Spirits. These colours have certain effects upon the various bodies of man and are related to the seven levels or planes of consciousness.

Colours as seen on the physical level are harsh and coarse compared to their appearance on the inner levels where they are of an inconceivable beauty and translucence. According to Bailey:

Indigo absorbs and is the colour of synthesis.
Green is the basis of the activity of nature and particularly related to the atmic plane. It both stimulates and heals.
Yellow harmonises and is the colour of completion and fruition, and the buddhic plane.
Blue is the colour of the higher mental plane.
Orange is the colour of the lower mental plane.
Rose is the colour of the astral plane.
Violet is the colour of ritual and the etheric levels.

She also points out that all colour healing should be handled from the mental plane, with the energies directed primarily at the mental body so that their effects will work from there to the astral and physical-etheric bodies. Colour treatment on the subtler planes is applied by the power of thought.

> Orange stimulates the action of the etheric body, removing conges-tion and increasing the flow of prana.
> Rose acts upon the nervous system by vitalising it. Increases the will to live, vitalises and removes depression.
> Green has a general healing effect. Useful for inflammatory states and fevers in particular.

HOMOEOPATHY AND RADIONICS

This is not the place to go into a dissertation on homoeopathy and radionics, but I simply wish to point out that healing through homoeopathic medicines has a very close affinity to the practice of radionics, and they can be employed in conjunction to great advantage. Every practitioner should have a *Materia Medica** that he can refer to in the course of remedy selection. What I want to do at this point is to draw some material from various esoteric sources which will serve as reference for practitioners and may prove useful in practice.

Rudolf Steiner contributed a great deal to our understanding of how certain remedies affect the inner bodies of man. The reader may find this information in *Spiritual Science and Medi-cine, Anthroposophical Approach to Medicine* and *Fundamentals of Therapy* the latter he co-authored with Dr. Ita Wegman. I am going to draw just one or two examples from these books as an indication of his insight into these matters.

Steiner combined metallic lead, honey and sugar to bring about harmony between the various subtle bodies in cases of sclerosis. Honey he said transfers the disintegrating effect of the astral body away from the physical-etheric levels.

Combining silicea, iron and sulphur provides those forces which bring balance to the energy systems in man when they are disturbed by migraine headaches.

*by William Boericke, M.D.
Also Tyler's *Homoeopathic Drug Pictures*, Clarke's *Dictionary of Practical Materia Medica* (3 volumes), Clarke's *Clinical Repertory*. All available at Health Science Press.

Iron pyrites are useful in the treatment of tracheitis and bronchitis.

Antimony carries the form-building forces of the human body into the blood and strengthens the forces that lead to the coagulation of blood. It weakens astral forces which give rise to eczema and is of use in treating typhoid fever.

Mercury and sulphur combined are useful in tracheitis and catarrh because of the effects upon the circulation and breathing processes. Hay fever, wherein the astral and etheric bodies are not properly coordinated is helped by the application of juices from fruits with leathery skins.

Steiner has some very remarkable things to say about fluorine which should interest a great many people, especially those who believe that they are doing their children a favour by giving the substance to them in tablet form. In the early 1920's before vested interests and the Establishment had found yet another way to legally poison the population and make money into the bargain, Steiner pointed out the following in respect to fluorine.

> Our teeth suck in fluorine. They are instruments of suction for that substance. Man needs fluorine in his organism in very minute amounts, and if deprived of its effects — here I must say something which will perhaps shock you — he becomes too clever. He acquires a degree of cleverness which almost destroys him. The fluorine dosage restores the necessary amount of stupidity, the mental dullness, which we need if we are to be human beings. . . . Man as it were disintegrates his teeth so that the fluorine action should not go beyond a certain point and make him dull. The interactions of cause and effect are very subtle here. The teeth become defective in order that the individual may not become too stupid. . . . Under certain circumstances we have need of the action of fluorine, in order not to become too clever. But we can injure ourselves by excess in this respect, and then our organic activity destroys and decays the teeth.

Excessive amounts of fluorine which is a residual poison cause all manner of organic lesions, not least of them mottling of the teeth. Promoters of fluoridated water never tire in their efforts to foist this form of medication on the public in the guise of preventative medicine, they never mention that their product is also waste from the aluminium industry and inorganic to boot. Natural fluorine has its place in the scheme of things, yet even it can cause problems if taken in excess. One can't help wondering what is behind this drive for mass medication with fluorine, are there forces that are bent on destroying the mental capabilities of masses of people while at the same time setting out to appear as public benefactors?

In the first chapter I mentioned a medical doctor by the name of B. Winter Gonin. He was one of the early pioneers to use radiesthesia in his practice, and he developed a remedy made up of various plant extracts called herbal hormone. In 1930 he published a booklet on the use of this remedy in which he pointed out that it was a very effective agent in the treatment of appendicitis, pleuritis, duodenitis, neuritis and useful as an antispasmodic. Tests showed that herbal hormone acted upon the reticulo-endothelial membranes, lymphoid tissue and the haematopoietic system to rapidly increase the number of leucocytes, phagocytes, the haemoglobin rate was also appreciably raised. A further point which will be of interest to the radionic practitioner is that Winter Gonin says:

> Loss of neuro-potential of the nervous system where leakage is to be found by the galvanometer is quickly restored, and in all cases where the aura shows "fracture" restitution takes place in situ.

Now Dr. Winter Gonin injected herbal hormone and radionic practitioners will not of course apply it in this way, but I know from experience that oral administration in tablet form or treatment by radionic projections will do much to help those patients who are suffering from 'leaks' in their aura. This remedy restores the electro-dynamic potential of the etheric body and it is for this reason that I have mentioned it here.

Another homoeopathic remedy that is said to have a profound restorative effect upon the etheric body is Moschus (Musk).

THE TWELVE TISSUE REMEDIES

Tissue salts are frequently called for when a practitioner combines homoeopathy with radionics, so I will list them here with a few of their basic indications. Fuller details can be gleaned from the Materia Medica but this list will serve as a quick reference to check through when selecting a remedy of this kind.

Calc Phos. (**Calcium Phosphate**) is present throughout all the body, and is an important constituent of the blood corpuscles, bones, teeth, gastric juices, and the connective tissues of the body. It is helpful when there is debility in digestion, also, since it is a tonic, it is valuable in convalescence, and for some types of anaemia. It should also be used for fractured bones.

Calc Sulph. (**Calcium Sulphate**) is a constituent of the blood and skin. It is therefore valuable in cases of suppuration of a heavy and persistent type, such as ulcers, abscesses, and heavy catarrh.

Calc Fluor. (**Calcium Fluoride**) is especially valuable for diseases affecting the surfaces of bones — the enamel of teeth and elastic fibres, particularly the muscles and the walls of arteries and veins. –? anthro or Arterio sclerosis.

Ferr Phos. (**Phosphate of Iron**) is a constituent of the red blood corpuscles, and is therefore one of the necessary remedies for anaemia, and in all cases where the blood lacks inorganic iron. It also strengthens the walls of the blood vessels. Again it is the remedy for high fevers and the early stages of inflammation from sudden injury or chill, which may bring on throbbing headaches, etc.

Kali Mur. (**Potassium Chloride**) is required whenever there is a thick white or grey coating of the tongue, since a deficiency of this salt produces an overflow of albumin to the tissues, resulting in catarrh or phlegm. It should be used in cases of croop, dysentery, bronchitis, pneumonia, diphtheria, etc.

Kali Phos. (**Potassium Phosphate**) is invaluable in the healing of nerve tissue, and therefore should be given in cases of brain and nerve depletion, which bring on such conditions as neurasthenia, excessive worrying, nervous exhaustion and depression. These may show themselves in dizziness, excessive sensitivity to noise, dysentery, etc.

Kali Sulph. (**Potassium Sulphate**) carries oxygen to the skin glands, and is therefore valuable in some skin diseases, since it assists in the opening of the pores and this in the increase of circulation. Those skin diseases that have slimy yellow secretions indicate the necessity for this salt. Also if the hair and skin are unhealthily oily, or the tongue has a slimy yellow coating.

Mag Phos. (**Magnesium Phosphate**) is invaluable for all sharp and spasmodic pains such as neuralgia, colic and painful menstruation. The relief is practically always immediate, and surprises those who have never used it. It is a nutrient of the white fibres of the motor nerves.

Nat Mur. (Sodium Chloride) is the distributor of water throughout the system, and is therefore useful in head colds and watery catarrhal symptoms. Also it checks the involuntary flow of tears or saliva.

Nat Phos. (Sodium Phosphate). Its action is to break up lactic acid and so liberate water in the system. For conditions of gastric fermentation, acidity and sour vomiting, rheumatic gouty ailments, gravel, etc.

Nat Sulph. (Sodium Sulphate) regulates water in the system. It is used for biliousness, jaundice, bilious headaches, kidney trouble, diabetes, and when the tongue has a dirty, brownish green coating.

Silicea (Silicon Oxide) is a constituent of the nerve sheaths and bone coverings, also of the hair, nails, and skin. It promotes suppuration and therefore helps to get rid of poisonous matter in the body. If there is catarrh with excessive thick discharge, debility, or much sweating, especially in the feet, this remedy should be used.

FLOWER REMEDIES AND GEMS

Like the Tissue Salts these remedies are often used in radionic practice and are either given orally or projected from ratio cards. The Bach Flower Remedies are probably the best known and their action is upon the mental and astral bodies of the patient. These are gentle remedies and can bring about no side-effects whatsoever. Once again I am going to include a full list which can be used for purposes of radiesthetic selection. Details of the conditions that these remedies are used for will be found in *The Bach Remedies Repertory*, *The Twelve Healers*, and *The Bach Flower Remedies.*

THE BACH FLOWER REMEDIES

Agrimony	Mimulus
Aspen	Mustard
Beech	Oak
Centaury	Olive
Cerato	Pine
Cherry Plum	Red Chestnut
Chestnut Bud	Rock Rose
Chicory	Rock Water
Clematis	Scleranthus
Crab Apple	Star of Bethlehem
Elm	Sweet Chestnut
Gentian	Vervain
Gorse	Vine
Heather	Walnut
Holly	Water Violet
Honeysuckle	White Chestnut
Hornbeam	Wild Oat
Impatiens	Wild Rose
Larch	Willow

Radiation Remedy, a combination of seven Bach flower remedies which Dr. Westlake and fellow researchers found effective as an antidote to the adverse effects of radio-active fallout.

One other Flower Remedy which must be listed is the one devised by the late Alick McInnes at Geddes, Nairn in Scotland. Its name is Exultation of Flowers, which comes in the form of liquid or ointment. This remedy is a combination of the etheric healing forces of some fifty or more flowers and it provides a powerful impetus to the healing forces of the body when taken orally or projected.

Gems too are another powerful healing agent. The best known proponent of this form of healing is Dr. A.K. Bhattacharrya of India. He lists the following gems and their related cosmic colours in this way.

Ruby	Red
Pearl	Orange

Coral	Yellow
Emerald	Green
Moonstone	Blue
Diamond	Indigo
Sapphire	Violet
Onyx	Ultra-violet
Cat's Eye	Infra-red

Details of this form of treatment are to be found in *Gem Therapy* by Dr. B. Bhattacharrya and *The Sceince of Cosmic Ray Therapy or Teletherapy* by the same author, both are revised and up-dated by Dr. A.K. Bhattacharrya to provide an excellent source of information for any radionic practitioner.

THE CHAKRAS AND RADIONIC TREATMENT

There is little that I need to touch upon here that has not been covered in my first two books on radionics. It is helpful perhaps to keep in mind the concept that all substance that goes into the makeup of the various bodies is capable of *intelligent response to stimulus*. The substance or attenuated matter of the chakras is even more sensitive and thus has a greater capacity to respond; this is an important factor to keep in mind when employing radionics to bring balance to those chakras that are either hypo or hyper active, or in any way damaged.

Flow must be kept in mind. Placing energy into a chakra is only the first step, it must be visualised to flow to the appropriate endocrine gland and on to the organ systems governed by the chakra and through the vehicles.

One system of radionic therapy says that the crown chakra should not be treated. This concept has no basis whatsoever in truth. It can be classified as idiosyncratic. The idea may have arisen because the crown chakra is ultimately the centre wherefrom the inner spiritual man governs the lower-self, however there is no bar in this that would preclude treatment of the crown chakra. The laying on of hands, the act of blessing a person, both involve, if done properly, the passing of invoked higher energies through the crown centre. It is the ideal point of entry to arouse the spiritual will-to-be in any individual.

In some instances practitioners will find that certain of the twenty-one minor chakras need treatment. Where indicated this may be carried out, but always remember that the major chakras govern the minor ones, and that proper balancing of the major will usually harmonise the functions of the minor centre or centres under its influence.

This then completes the section on considerations relative to radionic therapy; I have by no means covered everything because all radionic treatment is individually selected. The purpose of this chapter has been to list a number of items that might be useful, and to provide lists which can be checked radiesthetically when selecting treatment. I would like to close with a quotation from a book called The Chalice of the Heart, by Mary Gray, as it is appropriate to our theme.

> To heal a man, you must find the keynote of his vibration, and sound this with intensity, so as to reinforce his own chord and the vibratory song which is uniquely his.

SECTION FIVE

Other Dimensions

Today nobody can occupy a fixed position or find a fixed or stationary target. Electric technology excludes both possibilities.

Most people can still remember the time when fixed positions and fixed targets were taken for granted: the Establishment is still a nineteenth-century affair, entirely related to such assumptions. Our social, political and educational arrangements still assume goals and objectives as normal possibilities and aspirations.

In fact, however, a young doctor is as obsolete on the day he graduates as is any engineer.

Both have spent years acquiring long-packaged information data, while living in a total-field world of information mosaics that are moving at high speed.

Marshall McLuhan

CHAPTER TEN

Crossing the Interfaces

The quality of one's model of the universe is measured by how well it matches the real universe. There is no guarantee that one's current model does match the reality, no matter how certain one feels that it is a match of high quality.

The Human Biocomputer — John C. Lilley, M.D.

It seems that in order for the individual to be able to maintain some semblance of sanity and coherence of thought, he must operate from a series of fixed postures or beliefs. Without them the world takes on a peculiarly unstable appearance and rational behaviour is difficult. All of us to a greater or lesser degree base our approach to life on a fixed system of beliefs, this may be modified from time to time and remain flexible, or in extreme cases it takes on a rigidity that prevents the entrance of anything new that does not conform to its pattern.

Those of you who have read the books by Carlos Castaneda about his training as a sorcerer's apprentice to the Yaqui Indian don Juan, will perhaps recall that the old man spends the best part of ten years trying to get Castaneda to drop his view of the world and see it as it really is. He tells Castaneda that when a man is born he is handed a view of the world that gradually is reinforced to the point where it replaces reality. No one sees a tree, they only perceive their concept of what a tree is. The sorcerer seeks to show Castaneda how to see the real world, with techniques that are very reminiscent of those used by Zen Buddhist masters. When our view of the world drops away we experience satori or enlightenment wherein nothing stands between us and the world as it is.

All people to some extent then, are unable to see the world as it is. Professional training tends to intensify fixed positions and adherence to certain points of view which have been inculcated during training. This makes it very difficult for a doctor for example, to consider approaches to diagnosis and treatment which lie beyond his own belief system. Further, he is lead to believe that if modern medicine cannot take care of a problem then nothing else will, and he will stay with this belief no matter how much evidence he is offered to the contrary. There are of course exceptions to this rule, and one meets any number of doctors who are flexible in their approach to healing, and they accept that other disciplines are very effective in their own areas of application.

In the main though, most doctors and in fact others with very orthodox training, have great difficulty in coming to grips with the subjective aspects of radionics. Even Sir James Barr who used Abrams methods extensively in his practice, said of the latter's theory:

> But it must be clearly understood that we do not at this stage of our knowledge advance it as our own. We simply give it out of respect for the great genius to whose labor we directly owe the fact that we have been enabled to help many sick folk where otherwise we should have been powerless.

To come to grips with radionics it is necessary to adopt a whole different belief system, one in fact, that is larger than that held by orthodoxy. Bearing this in mind, you will appreciate that radionics can only widen your view of the world and not in any way diminish it. As far as science is concerned a dried spot of blood is of little or no clinical use whatsoever. The radionic practitioner holds a different view which is reflected in the following passage from *Abrams' Methods of Diagnosis and Treatment* by Sir James Barr.

> Dr. Abrams, on the strength of the generally accepted electronic theory of matter, originated the idea that dried blood radiated electronic energy; that this energy varied as regards vibration-characteristics according to whether the blood was healthy or diseased; and that different kinds of disease were characterised by different kinds of radiated energy.

Having perhaps agreed that there might be some truth in this, the doctor is now faced with diagnosis at a distance. Diagnosis with the patient linked physically to the instrument is one thing, to claim it can be done through the blood spot when the patient is absent is a whole new concept which once again requires flexibility of beliefs. Even Abrams towards the end discovered that he could identify energies coming from a patient at a distance of one mile. It took Ruth Drown to push distance as a factor to one side and demonstrate that it made no difference where the patient was when diagnosis, or for that matter treatment, was carried out.

Drown saw quite clearly that a new era in healing had opened up, and in 1939 she wrote:

> The age of the healing art wherein the patient was given remedies and chemicals of the earht and water has now advanced another step, and has entered into the air cycle — conforming to the advent of the radio, television and wireless.

This is an example of a person working from a flexible and not a fixed position. I am sure Marshall McLuhan would have found in Ruth Drown a true twentieth-century exponent of electric technology; perhaps she was even more than that, recognising and making use of the electrical forces of space, the fohat of Theosophy or the prana of Indian tradition, as she did. Perhaps Drown was a pioneer exponent of the twenty-first century technology, which will no doubt reveal aspects of electrical phenomena that are incomprehensible to us at this point in time.

Again and again in radionics the investigating doctor is faced with new beliefs, most of which are not subscribed to by orthodoxy. The only recognisable constant he is going to come across is that pathological states go by the same name in radionics as they do in medicine. Mumps is mumps whatever your approach to healing may be, however in radionics the causative factor may prove to be different, the viral aspect being only a part of the picture. Physical anatomy too will be the same, but here again there is the far more important subtle anatomy; the emphasis is upon the subjective, and not the gross objectivity of organ systems. Remedies and treatment often seem peculiar to the orthodox mind as well, so that overall if a doctor hopes to come to any understanding of radionics he must be capable of holding orthodox beliefs in abeyance until he has come to see the basic principles of this approach to healing have their own validity based on their own reality. The same of course would apply to osteopaths, chiropractors and naturopaths, although by and large they generally have less difficulty in relating to such concepts.

Drown was very perceptive when she said of radionic practice:

When we realize that we are dealing with this Life-Force, it teaches us about ourselves.

One thing is certain, no person who deals with the Life-Force for any length of time, can maintain a fixed position within a rigid belief system, because this force works upon the individual if he will allow it to and presents to the perceptive observer a veritable kaleidoscope of possibilities and potential. By its very nature it opens the individual to its expansive rhythmic flow, and as more is learned about it more is known about the Self. Under such conditions it soon becomes apparent that fixed positions and static belief systems are not allied to life but opposed to it.

The model of reality that orthodox medicine is based on is obviously a functional, mechanistic one. When radionics is brought into the realm of medicine by the individual doctor it will enfold his belief system, soften its hard edges and supply other dimensions to it which will add depth to his capacity to understand and heal that he has never before experienced. Of the Tao it is said:

> It blunts sharpness,
> Resolves tangles;
> It tempers light,
> Subdues turmoil.

Perhaps we should add; knowing it, precludes the holding of any fixed position; change is a universal constant and a particularly important one in any field of healing.

One of the first things the Life-force teaches any practitioner is that he must render himself effective. By this is meant that he:

The healer must understand also how to radiate, for the radiation of the soul will stimulate to activity the soul of the one to be healed and the healing process will be set in motion; the radiation of the mind will illumine the other mind and polarise the will of the patient; the radiation of his astral body, controlled and selfless, will impose a rhythm upon the agitation of the patient's astral body, and so enable the patient to take right action, whilst the radiation of the vital body, working through the splenic centre, will aid in organising the patient's force-body and so facilitate the work of healing. Therefore, the healer has the duty of rendering himself effective, and according to what he is, so will be the effect upon the patient.

How does a practitioner then, render himself effective? First he accumulates knowledge and while doing so he purifies first his motives and then his vehicles of manifestation through prayer, meditation, proper diet and a balanced life-style. He renders himself magnetic and his bodies are so tuned to their Source, that all who touch upon his consciousness receive healing. He keeps in mind that his life is a continuum flowing through cycles of what we call life and death, and he knows that every day is a day of preparation and opportunity. Now is the eternal point of power, the Christ within, and he learns to hold his consciousness at that point at all times. It is never too late nor too early to bring the personality into synchronised alignment with the soul, for that is an important milestone along the path of its destiny. If a pateint should reach out in thought towards the practitioner, or pick up the phone to call, or sit down to write a letter asking for help, and that practitioner's consciousness is focussed in his soul, the healing process will immediately be initiated. If you wonder about this I can assure you that there is no shortage of anecdotes in which a person has written for help, and due to pressure of work the practitioner has left the letter unopened for a day or two, only to have the patient call and say, "I don't know what you've done, but I feel marvellous". If the practitioner's consciousness is focussed deep within himself, instantaneous healings may occur, even in people who do not know of him, yet are reaching out in prayer for help. This is not taught in medical schools, nor colleges of chiropractic or osteopathy, nor in radionic training for that matter, but it does point out the need for the practitioner to pay attention to how he polarises his consciousness throughout the day. In his book *The High Walk of Discipleship* Eugene Cosgrove wrote:

> There is another spiritual effective and of planetary importance. It should therefore be anchored deep in the heart of the physician of the soul. It lies in the subjective existence of the vast reservoirs of spiritual power centred in and around the Healing Christ. Surely a plus factor of the highest significance for anyone who essays the power to heal!

That reservoir of healing power is always present, always available; the practitioner has to learn to link his own thoughtform of healing to it. I suppose that if this power could be confined in some kind of algebraic or mathematical formula, then science and medicine might concede its existence. However this is not the case, nor is it ever likely to be, and the doctor who contemplates the use of radionics in his practice or as an investigatory tool, will learn in time that at some point in his past, he has made a vow to serve in the field of healing, and that his medical education is but a very small part of the basic training he will undergo through many lifetimes. Radionics is the door, the key if you like, that will ease him into a wider understanding of the processes of disease and the implementation of wholeness, that will eradicate imbalances in a sure and lasting way. Healing is not the endless use of drugs but a true understanding of consciousness. Every individual who has committed himself to serve as a healer, will at some time or another pass through the various disciplines that man has to offer, for they provide the ground upon which every healer must firmly place his feet. Cosgrove says:

> Every spiritual healer is by the divine right of his own soul a member of the church of the Healing Christ, and participates to his measure in the function of The Christ as the healer of healers. Such a healer

is ordained of his own soul to the healing ministry. He needs no other ordination, nor can any other ordination add to (or take from) his power to heal.

With this in mind, and the directive to render oneself effective, we can stop for a moment to consider the importance of the magnetic purity of the practitioner. Firstly a radiant, clear set of bodies allows the practitioner to properly register what is wrong with the patient; and secondly, if his mental, astral and etheric vehicles are fully charged with the vital forces, his sensitivity which is especially needed in any radiesthetic work, will be at full power. Baron Von Reichenbach who experimented with pendulums and the relationship of their actions to the odic force, found that sensitives who normally carried a high charge of the Life-Force in their vital body could use the pendulum to better effect than people who did not. In his book under the heading 'Motive Power of the Aura' the following appears:

Pendulum Movements: In order to dissipate popular errors and superstitions connected with the pendulum, Reichenbach describes in his Aphorisms, how he constructed a small pendulum free to move under a glass shade which cut off the influence of air-currents, but which left a small aperture at the top through which a finger could be laid on the motionless portion of a long string wound round a windlass with a little ball of lead suspended at the free end of the string. He found that he himself and all ordinary persons could produce no movements whatsoever by touching the fixed end of the string.

He was about to do away with his apparatus, thinking he had effectually disproved a source of popular superstition, when he chanced to ask a high-sensitive to lay his finger at the touch-point. Decided and unmistakable swinging of the pendulum resulted. Further experiments convinced him that all sensitives, and sensitives alone, possessed this power, the length of the oscillation in the pendulum depending on the degree of sensitiveness, low, medium or high, in the operator, and also the state of the operator's health. He gives further details as follows:

If the right hand of the sensitive produce 8-line oscillations, and another right hand be laid upon it, diffusing like od, the oscillations are increased to 12-lines. If a left hand be laid on the operator's right, the motion of the pendulum at once ceases. If odically negative matter, such as selenium, sulphur, charcoal, etc., be placed in the operator's left, the oscillations increase; if the same be done with odically positive matter, such as iron, copper, tin, lead, the pendulum stands still at once.

If the operator has a watch, a key, or coins in his pocket, he is unfitted thereby to produce oscillations, no matter how high his degree of sensitivity. On one occasion I made an operator who had got rid of all metals on his person and produce 10-line oscillations, pull on his boots with iron nails in the soles, and his pendulum came to a standstill at once.

The negative od takes its course from the sensitive's hand along the cord, which should not be too fine, and down to the plummet, which I had made 6 oz. in weight, diffuses a visible glow along the cord and around the plummet, is odically luminous in the dark chamber, and produces rectilinear oscillations proportionate in length to the amount of od discharged.

In the Rae Magneto-Geometric Analyser a layer of rubber impregnated with minute magnetized filings sits beneath the analysis and treatment charts, this serves to augment the odic field of the operator, and is thought to help cut out interference from the conscious mind during diagnostic work.

Sensitivity then is a vital part of radiesthetic work, and this can be improved and maintained at a high pitch if the practitioner is prepared to understand what is involved, and to act upon it. One of the finest papers ever delivered on the radiesthetic sense was given at a conference in 1972 by Dr. Aubrey Westlake. It is included as a part of this chapter because the information it contains should be grasped by any practitioner who wishes to take up radionics, in order that he may know what he is about when making a diagnosis on subjective levels.

THE ROLE AND SCOPE OF THE RADIESTHETIC FACULTY IN THE MODERN WORLD*

It is I believe salutary to step back, so to speak, from time to time and survey the whole field of study and activities in which we as the Society of Dowsers are engaged, to see what we have accomplished, what we are doing at present, and what should be our contribution to the future.

The last time I made an attempt to do this was in 1955, when at the Congress that year I gave, perhaps rashly, a paper on the

*A lecture given at the Congress of the British Society of Dowsers held at Malvern, 5th May, 1972. Copies of this lecture and 'The Scope and Limitations of Radiesthetic Investigation' by Malcolm Rae are included together in booklet form. Available from Magneto-Geometric Applications. Price 50p inc. postage.

Future of Radiesthesia, and in the light of what has in fact happened I am glad to see I was not too bad a prophet.

My reason for attempting a similar survey 17 years later, under the present title, is because I believe we have still not realized the full significance of what we in the B.S.D. have banded together to practise and promote in these modern times.

It is still my belief, even more so than in 1955, that we have a great contribution to make, a contribution much greater than we envisage or imagine, as we are in fact in possession of a vital key which could unlock many doors of apparently insoluble modern problems, especially that of world-wide pollution in its many forms.

This key is the Radiesthetic Faculty, and the development of its full potentialities and their practical use and application which go far beyond the traditional finding of water, mineral ores and oil.

But let us start at the beginning.

The phenomenon of Dowsing is very ancient. Neolithic man probably knew all about its practical use especially for sacred structures, and the ancient Egyptians certainly did; but it was not until A.D. 1240 that we have any reference in European writings, and the first reference in England was in 1638 in a book written in Latin by Robert Fludd entitled *Philosophic Moysayko,* followed next year by a certain Gabriel Platts who wrote abour "A Discovery of Subterraneall Treasure. The operation with the Virgula Divina is thus to be performed — I cut a rod of Hassel, I tied it to my staff in the middle with a strong thread so that it did hang even, and carried it up and downe the mountaines and it guided me to a veine of lead ore".* Dowsing during these times was always regarded as something mysterious, even magical and certainly having no rational explanation, and the movement of the rod attributable to either God or the Devil, or some baser spirits.

Since that date although dowsing was well known both on the Continent and in this country it was not until the end of the 19th century that any systematic study was made of it, but in 1897 Prof. William Barrett, F.R.S., published a paper in the Proceedings of the Society for Psychical Research entitled "On the so-called Divining Rod or Virgula Divina — a scientific and historical research as to the existence and practical value of a peculiar human faculty, unrecognized by science, locally known as dowsing, with letters from 208 correspondents describing 140 cases of water-finding by 46 professionals and 38 amateur dowsers in 256 localities". And he made a further contribution to the Proceedings in 1900 "On the so-called Divining Rod — a psycho-physical research on a peculiar faculty

---

*There is a note in the B.M. copy that "The author of this book died of meer want in ye year 1646 in London — he was a rare man for feats of husbandry, and chemistry, etc".

alleged to exist in certain persons locally known as dowsers, together with appendices by Ernest Westlake [my father] on the geological aspects of dowsing". The role and scope at this time were almost entirely confined to water and mineral ore dowsing, but the publication of these papers made dowsing for the first time a legitimate subject for scientific study. Subsequently they were added to and made into book form and published in 1926 under the title *The Divining Rod*.

The next milestone in England was the inauguration of the B.S.D. in 1933, and if you look at early numbers of the Journal you will see that the first object of the newly formed society was "to encourage the study of all matters connected with the perception of radiation by the human organism with or without instruments". Very wisely the founders, of whom Col. Bell was the leading spirit, did not define what was meant or included under the phrase "the perception of radiation", but made the scope of the society as wide and inclusive as possible. I am sure that this has enabled the B.S.D. to have such success as it has had during the 39 years of its existence, as it has thankfully remained undifferentiated and has not become specialized.

Fortunately the founders also recognized at the beginning that the Society was not just concerned with finding water or mineral deposits, but with "all matter connected with the perception of radiation by the human organism" which, in other words, is what I mean by the title of this lecture, "The role and scope of the radiesthetic faculty", as the phenomenon of all forms and aspects of dowsing are completely dependent on the radiesthetic faculty and its right and proper functioning. Their foresight is of considerable importance as it has made possible developments which I regard as crucial in view of the intractable problems of the modern world.

At the beginning the Society and its members were naturally mainly concerned with the traditional form of this perception in the phenomena of Rhabdomancy — to use the old term for dowsing — which is defined "as the use of the divining rod especially for discovering subterranean water or ore".

But the early days of the Society were filled with controversy between those who believed dowsing was purely a physical phenomena and could be explained in terms of modern physics, particularly electro-magnetism, and those who held it to be primarily a psychic phenomena. The late Mr. Maby, that indefatigable researcher, was a great advocate of the physical school of thought and indeed he said that once one departed from the physical "all is chaos, confusion, subjectivity and nonsense". But he did a great service to dowsing in insisting on the physical aspect which he set out in his book *The Physics of the Divining Rod* published in 1949; as it cleared the decks, so to speak. For it was essential first to determine the nature and extent of this physical aspect before it was possible to make a real advance in what may be regarded as the true idiom of the subject.

Maby's mistake was not in what he affirmed but in what he denied, in thinking that because the radiesthetic faculty could detect physical radiations that anything else belonged to what he called divination and was not dowsing as he understood it and its exploration necessarily unscientific and subjective. At the time he had a good deal of justification for his views, as the techniques and the required instruments to explore the supersensible side were not understood and thus not used, even though they could probably have been available.

But it was gradually realized, and by no less authority than Sir William Barrett, that the attempt to account for dowsing on physical grounds alone must be abandoned; and indeed it is fortunate, for if physical radiesthesia were indeed all, we should be in sight of the end of dowsing for water, minerals and oil, as it is abundantly clear that in the purely material field the dowser will probably be superseded by the development of ultra sensitive instruments capable of picking up and analysing all material radiations.

Nevertheless apart from Maby's and Franklin's research works little progress had been made by 1953 in other fundamental research, so much so that such an accomplished dowser as the late Major Pogson, when asked whether there had been any major advance in technique and results in the last 30 years, said he was bound to admit there had been none.

Round about this time, as I recount in the *Pattern of Health*, I met Mr. W.O. Wood and had a remarkable association with him until his death in the autumn of 1957. I found that he was all out for action, as he was clear that if ever we were going to solve the mystery of radiesthesia, we should have to enlarge and reorientate our ideas and concepts in a very vital and fundamental way. The physical and materialistic outlook is not enough. It is valid as far as it goes, as we have seen in Maby's work for example, but beyond that is a vast world which is at once scientific and religious and can only be understood in the light of "spiritual science", to use Rudolf Steiner's term.

The action he was after, in the light of this, he finally instituted in the winter of 1954-55 during an intense cold spell, and proved to be an exploration in depth of the radiesthetic technique now called Q & A, which I will consider more fully later on.

The main outcome of this work apart from its intrinsic value was that it brought him recognition as a sound researcher and he was asked to give the lecture following the Annual General Meeting of the B.S.D. in 1955. He chose as his subject "Observations on Some Problems facing the Society". As an outside observer he said he had a feeling for some time that the B.S.D. was not realizing its potentials or possibilities and had fallen into a state of scientific stagnation. Let me quote this passage from his lecture:

"The most important feature is the dowser's apparent un-
willingness to tackle the full scope of the gift of sensitivity, and
his tendency to restrict his thoughts to what has been described
as the hewing of wood and the drawing of water. The thinking
public are now well aware that the range of sensitivity cannot thus
be circumscribed. The problems facing mankind are greater than
the locating of wells and matching of remedies — plumbing and
plastering, so to speak — and we have to come to grips with the
issues of our times and face realities as they are. It is necessary
that the sights of the dowser be raised in line with those of science
and philosophy — so a problem is presented: whether the urgency
and magnitude of the factors facing man do not force upon the
dowser the choice between widening the scope of his activities, or
rejection as having failed to provide for the full flowering of the
gift entrusted to him — for the principles the dowsers seek are
known to others, who seek in turn the means of proving them.
The dowser has the means of proving them, but appears these
days to be blind to the principles."

But there was already at this time one important exception, viz.,
in the field of medical dowsing, or radiesthesia as it came to be
known from its French origin.

Starting as far back as the turn of the century, radiesthesia had
already been practised successfully by many French priests, notably
the Abbés Bouley and Mermet, and by other accomplished technicians
such as Turrene, Lesourd, Bovis and many others.

Knowledge of all this promising work came, in due course, to
England, and six years after the founding of the B.S.D., the Medical
Society for the Study of Radiesthesia was started in 1939 by Dr.
Guyon Richards. He gathered round him a remarkable group of
qualified medical men as well as some outstanding lay members. The
Society remained very alive and active for many years in spite of the
loss of its founder Dr. Guyon Richards in 1946, followed by six
others of the original group between then and 1952. Some years
later it shed its lay associate members, since when, while still alive,
it has ceased to be active.

Fortunately one member of the original group — Dr. George
Laurence — has not only carried on and is still with us, but during
the fifties and sixties developed and worked out a technique of
diagnosis and treatment arising from clinical research work and
assessment which is now known as Psionic Medicine embracing,
among other things, McDonagh's Unitary Theory of Disease and
Hahnemann's Theory of Chronic Disease, the latest work on DNA
and RNA, and some aspects of Steiner's Spiritual Science, but all
depending on the functioning of the radiesthetic faculty. In 1969
the Psionic Medical Society was formed with both medical and
lay membership, to foster and promote this new approach to the

science and art of healing, which discovers, by the use of the radies-thetic faculty, the really basic cause or causes lying at the root of disorder or disease, and then treats these by radiesthetically indicated homoeopathic remedies — real creative medicine. In this it has been gratifyingly successful, and with a technique of the simplest — a pendulum, a diagnostic chart, and actual witnesses, these latter to give greater reliability to the readings.

So in this field there has been much research and definite basic progress thanks to the full use of the radiesthetic faculty.

But medical dowsing also had an influx from a completely different source, this time from America, in the work of Dr. Albert Abrams whom Sir James Barr described as "by far the greatest genius the medical profession has produced for half a century". He produced, after an incredible amount of research and fortuitous good luck, his famous "Box", from which was developed in due course the Drown diagnostic and treatment instruments, and later those of de la Warr, which later in turn gave birth to Radionics — instrumental radiesthe-sia — and the Radionic Association formed in 1943 "to assist scientific investigation, and the propagation of its findings". Unfor-tunately as had happened with straightforward water divining, under-standing was badly hampered by the desire to explain the phenomena in terms of orthodox physics and to get the approval of orthodox science, and even when later the Association was re-formed as a breakaway from the de la Warr set-up, and took a new lease of life, it was, in its early days, still bogged down in and with gadgets and gadgetry, and the true nature of the phenomena and this form of diagnosis and healing largely missed. But gradually the unique role of the radiesthetic faculty has been recognized as will be clear when we come to the technique of Q & A.

But apart from this development of medical dowsing in its two forms of radiesthesia and radionics there seemed to be a state of relative stagnation on the dowsing front and wider implications of Wood's warnings remained unheeded.

It appeared to me at this time that the important thing which must be done was to swtich our attention from the mechanics of dowsing to the one factor essential to the phenomena however it was operated, viz., the dowsing faculty; and so in 1959, at the Congress held in July, I read a paper entitled "The Radiesthetic Faculty" which was an attemtp to understand the essential nature and function of this mysterious sense.

I do not propose now to go over my findings which in any case you can find in Chap. XII of the *Pattern of Health*, and my later thoughts on the subject in Chap. XVI of *Life Threatened*, but let me quote this summary:

"I believe that the rediscovery of the radiesthetic faculty in these modern times is not fortuitous, but that it has been vouch-

safed to us by Providence to enable us to cope with the difficult
and dangerous stage in human development which lies immediately
ahead, for it gives indirect access to the supersensible world, more
particularly to the etheric, this raising our level of consciousness
and extending our awareness and knowledge. The faculty should
be regarded as a special and peculiar sense halfway between our
ordinary physical senses which apprehend the material world,
and our to-be-developed future occult senses which, in due course,
will apprehend the supersensible world direct."

"It is moreover a faculty which can operate on various levels,
particularly the subconscious or Huna Low Self level, but also on the
superconscious or Huna High Self level and higher ones still, according
to the requirements of the situation and the training, discipline and
knowledgableness of the operator. This will I hope become clear
when we come to discuss Q & A.

In my book *Life Threatened*, written some years later, I discussed
again what I thought was the modus operandi of the faculty and
suggested, I imagined with good reason, that the proprioceptive
nervous system was directly involved, but further work would suggest
that this was erroneous and that the working sequence is — etheric
formative forces — > red blood cells — > the circulatory blood — >
the autonomic nervous system — > voluntary muscles — > the movement of the pendulum.

This said, let us go back to Wood's lecture. If he at that time felt
so strongly that the problems of 1955 needed "the full scope of the
dowser's sensitivity", to use his own words, the need must be very
much greater today with the vast and additional problems of 1972.
Let us consider some of those to which it would appear we can make
a very special and probably unique contribution to their understanding
and solution in these modern times and one moreover now acceptable, if recent books like Arthur Koestler's *The Roots of Coincidence*
and Edward Russell's *Design for Destiny* are any indication of public
interest and concern. Here is a tentative list, but one which can and
doubtless will be added to:

1. The search for water, oil and mineral deposits. This is the
well-known traditional field of dowsing and has in fact been, and
still is, well covered though not as much as it should be by both
professional and amateur dowsers.
2. Archaeological exploration. A more limited field at present
but of considerable and increasing importance for historical
research and the recovery of vanished prehistoric remains.
3. Architectural uses, such as site dowsing, in which must be
included detection of harmful earth rays and detection of cavities,
pipes and drains etc. No dwelling should be built until the site has
been properly dowsed. Also the actual building materials are

important, and also the substances used in the furniture; steel, for example, dulls the brain — it is a mineral hypnotic.

4.   The locating of law breakers and criminals, missing persons, dead bodies, and lost or buried property and money. Increasingly important with the great increase in crime of late years. Should be used far more than it is in civil and criminal cases needing such aid.

5.   Agricultural and horticultural uses. In such things as the determination of optimum soil conditions, seed fertility and germination, plant health, and of good husbandry in general including the value of all additives both organic and inorganic. Determination of quality, aliveness and wholesomeness in all foods whether natural, manufactured, processed, or artificial and synthetic.

6.   Personality assessment, by measurement of "brain radiation" as discovered and used by Dr. Oscar Brunler. It has manifold uses, educationally and industrially, in estimation of talents, aptitudes, personality problems and mental potential, etc.

7.   Medical and Veterinary application. Apart from water divining, medicine has received more radiesthetic attention as I have already pointed out, but there are still innumerable problems to solve, and the only answer to many of them is in Psionic Medicine both diagnostically and theraputically. Already enough is known to change the whole pattern of medical treatment but the public is being deprived by entrenched orthodoxy of this help and knowledge and of what can be done both curatively and prophylactically.

In veterinary practice, if used more extensively it would undoubtedly help to prevent the gradual deterioration of vitality, stamina and resistance in farm and domestic animals.

8.   Homoeopathy. The introduction of radiesthesia into the practice of homoeopathy would unquestionably mean a great revival in homoeopathic medicine, either as its own speciality or more sensibly in the form of a comprehensive medicine such as Psionic Medicine. Radiesthesia in this context solves the vexed and difficult question of remedy selection and potency.

9.   Here we come to our modern dilemma — the whole vast problem of pollution and contamination particularly in its subtle and more intangible aspects of the present ubiquitous paratoxic environment in which we all now have to live or exist.

Out of the innumerable toxic factors let me mention two groups, firstly, the low level radio-activity of Tritium (a radioactive isotope of hydrogen 3H) and Carbon 14, also radio-active, as expounded so brilliantly by David Rawson in his monograph *Radiation and Nuclear Homoeopathy*. The menace from these two began to be serious in 1954 and is steadily increasing thanks

to the thermonuclear testings and the so-called peaceful use of
atomic energy. The menace arises from the fact that in every
hydrological and carbon cycle in Nature these radio-active isotopes
are now present, even in the hydrogen bonds which hold together
the intricate helical structure of DNA and RNA in our bodies – a
truly frightening thought.

Secondly the increasing toxic menace of Lead, Mercury and
Cadmium in our ordinary encironment, in human and animal
bodies, and in the rivers, seas and oceans of the world.

Radiesthesia can be of inestimable value in giving us the
knowledge and techniques of how to detect and deal with the
subtle poisoning effects of all the polluting factors, for as Dr.
Weinberg, Head of the Oakridge Atomic Energy Establishment
– the Harwell of America – said publicly: "The problems at one
rad are not amenable to the scientific method. Other approaches
are necessary." He tables those questions which are beyond investigation with present assay methods as "trans-scientific."

Psionic medicine already provides one of these "other
approaches" for dealing with the effects in humans and animals;
and doubtless other approaches, using the radiesthetic faculty to
discover them, will also be forthcoming.

10.   And so to the last in our list – Question and Answer. Q & A.
In which the operator must learn to use faculties of intellect and
intuition, applying either at will and never confusing them – the
intellect for the formulation of questions and the evaluation of
answers, and the intuition, using the radiesthetic faculty, to
obtain the truth. Q & A is eminently the instrument of scientific
radiesthetic research.

This I regard as the most important use of the radiesthetic
faculty as it provides a bridge between two worlds – the sensible
and the supersensible.

The elements of seeking and finding are of course inherent in all
radiesthetic and dowsing work, but it is only in Q & A that they become
a deliberate technique, and there is conscious "asking".

As far as I know the first recorded use of the radiesthetic faculty
in this way for deliberate research was carried out in 1956 by the
group whose activities I recorded in my book *Pattern of Health*.
The success of the group was undoubtedly largely due, in the first
place, to Mr. Wood whom I described as "an ideal question-master":
"His skill at this was quite remarkable, as he had exceptional flair for
framing precise and correct wording of the question, and following
it up with exactly the right supplementaries. He had a quick and
agile mind, yet at the same time it was balanced and usually under
the control of his highly informed reason. An ideal combination. "In
the second place success was due to the two sensitives who were
sufficiently developed to be able to work on the levels required.

Those of you who have read the *Pattern of Health*, particularly the chapter in question, will know the invaluable insights which were vouchsafed us at this time particularly in regard to the levels of consciousness on which the radiesthetic faculty operates, and the fact that "pattern" appeared to be of great importance in this work, which in this instance emerged in the seven healing patterns, of which the first three — the Diamond, the Celtic Cross and the Star of Bethlehem — gave such remarkable theraputic results. The conditions governing legitimate use of Q & A were also worked out.

But there the matter rested and has remained dormant for some years now, as with the death of Mr. Wood in 1957 the group dispersed and no further group research was done.

Just recently however it has blossomed forth again in an enhanced form in the work of two talented researchers in the radionic and radiesthetic fields of study.

The first is Mrs Jane Wilcox who most fortunately was able to draw on the experience and informed advice of Major Blythe Praeger (one of the members of the original group) and who proved to be a very apt pupil. So much so that at the recent Conference of the Association in March this year she gave the closing lecture entitled "Question and Answer", with the intriguing sub-title of "A Bridge Between Two Worlds". This was cast in the form of query and answer, her husband asking the questions. This proved to be an outstanding contribution. All who were fortunate enough to hear it felt that here was a great advance in our understanding of the role and scope of the radiesthetic faculty.

What impressed me particularly was that her own investigation of the technique confirmed our original findings, but also produced some most important additions; for example she started off originally simply to improve the reliability of her own radionic healing work but found, to quote her:

"That the whole process of the art of Q & A is a vastly larger subject than a means of obtaining specific information in any one specialized field. I see it as a means of integrating the personality and of learning how to construct a bridge between the conscious and unconscious worlds in relation to life as a whole. In short that Q & A can be used as a process of self-development.

Understanding and integrating herself as a personality she found necessitated the awareness of her subconscious — the Low Self in Huna philosophy — that as it can be a good servant but a bad master, it had to be properly instructed and disciplined, otherwise it gave the answer that it thought the conscious self wanted, or else played up, or in certain instances gave false answers, for unconscious emotional reasons.

But equally and more importantly it meant a recognition and

realization of the existence of the super-conscious or Huna High Self, how to contact it and how to differentiate between the roles and functions of the two selves, as well as the relationship of the conscious or Middle Self to the other two, and the need for the acquisition above all else, in this relationship, of clear and responsible thinking.

The construction of the "bridge" required:-

1.   A mode and code of communication i.e. the movements of the pendulum and their interpretation.

2.   The nature and formulation of the questions to be asked which requires

(a)   finding out in any given case whether the question is legitimate e.g. idle curiosity is out, questions about the future, and inadequate formulation due to insufficient knowledge.

(b)   if it is legitimate, the need for clear and precise thinking based on adequate knowledge so that there is no ambiguity or double meaning which in its turn means

(c)   finding the right word or words to exactly express the thought. This requires a large vocabulary, and English with its richness of language and abundant synonyms is ideal for this purpose, and the book which is essential is Roget's Thesaurus; and to help in this task of exact selection, Q & A can be legitimately used.

3.   The answer then requires intellectual assessment as to whether it makes sense or not, if it does this will lead to other questions and the elucidation of the given problem. Or it may make nonsense or there may be no answer at all. If this latter, Mrs Wilcox says that at the beginning she looks for interfering emanations usually paranormal, but gradually came to realize this was too facile an interpretation and that it meant something was to be learnt, that, what she called the "teaching element" of the High Self was trying to draw her attention to something important and thereby broaden her ability to understand the truth. She found in this situation she had to ask four questions.

(a)   Am I allowed to ask this question?

(b)   Am I asking the wrong question?

(c)   Are 'You' trying to teach me something?

(d)   Do I need to ask a subsidiary question before you can answer me?

4.   It is necessary to realize that the answer may come from two levels, from the subconscious or the superconscious. Apart from the nature of the content of the answers there is an essential difference which one comes to recognize — the answer from the superconscious sources have, to quote Mrs Wilcox: "an authenticity and simplicity of quality which just does have a true ring about it". But on this level ask and ye shall receive holds good, but you *must* ask; but clarity of thought in framing questions is a must —

neither source can answer muddled questions.

5.   Finally the most vital realization of all is, according to Mrs Wilcox, "that no help will be forthcoming unless and until one has first done one's very best to answer the question by utilizing one's natural gifts and faculties".

The second researcher in this field is Mr. Malcolm Rae who interestingly enough came to Radionics from a life of wide experience both in commerce and business. But being a very practical and inventive type he thought at first that advance would come from improved and more sophisticated radionic instruments, and in fact he produced a very successful 40 dial one. But he soon came to see that it was not so much this that was wanted, as an improved human operator whose essential requisites are:

1. That he or she is a seeker after truth
2. Has a trained and disciplined intellect
3. Has a wide and varied knowledge
4. Has a well developed and trained radiesthetic faculty.
5. Has a simple instrumental technique

and that the research undertaken should be based on actual problems confronting the investigator whether in medical work or indeed in all the other fields already mentioned.

I find myself in a difficulty in trying to record his work, for as more supersensible knowledge has come through it is constantly changing both in form and content in order to incorporate the additional truth revealed. Such advances come about as a result of pegging away at the cases he is treating which do not respond to treatment, and thus the endeavour to find out why; what has been missed; had there been a wrong interpretation; or does the problem require looking at from a new angle?

But in this way a truer and truer pattern of healing has begun to emerge with proportionally less and less failures. This however has required a very flexible approach and the rethinking of a number of things, e.g. the real nature of those mysterious radionic rates, as well as many other things apparently accepted as gospel truth.

In February this year he gave a paper to the Medical Society for the Study of Radiesthesia entitled *Radiesthesia and Thought* which is an excellent example of how, employing the radiesthetic faculty in the technique of Q & A, it can be used as the instrument par excellence in basic scientific radiesthetic research.

He found that one of the first essentials is to distinguish between truth, i.e. facts, and opinion, and he suggests that if the usual intellectual assessment of relative truth is used it is very difficult to do this, but using radiesthetic assessment the task is far more sure and conclusive. This he found could be done by a suitable designed truth chart on a base of magnetic rubber, which latter tends to reduce the interference of the intellect.

Working with this and Q & A it has been possible to determine certain fundamental axioms such as, and I quote Malcolm Rae: "Everything in the universe, as far as I know, consists of a system of energies operating within boundaries. The boundaries describe structure and the energies describe functioning within the structure."

This led to the concept, and I quote again:

"Any deviation from the planned function of anything in the universe is caused by an alteration in the pattern of boundaries and energies. Any detrimental deviation is due to the displacement of a boundary, and a displaced boundary becomes a barrier. The introduction of a barrier into a system of boundaries and energy flows tends to turn all boundaries into barriers and all energies into stresses.

"As the radiesthetic faculty would appear to detect boundaries and/or barriers it can therefore be used to measure the difference between a boundary and a barrier and this would represent the degree of deviation from normality or health."

This difference or deviation can be expressed in mathematical terms in what would appear to be sets of co-ordinates of a very complex nature, and in the case of Man involving six sets in the given frame of reference which can be determined radiesthetically in detail, and which describes all facets of Man in his environment.

This introduction of mathematics is very interesting for as Canon Galzeswki in a paper entitled "The Human Field in Medical Problems" said, and I quote:

"In 1946 Prof. Mayer Ibach from the medical faculty of Hamburg University came to see me and spent five hours in discussion, insisting that maths should somehow be introduced into medical problems. He was at that time, as he said to me, writing a history of medicine, and that whenever maths was used in this branch of knowledge medicine was rapidly developing, and has declined in its absence. It was for both of us a problem how this could be effected properly."

Malcolm Rae has it seems provided an answer.

These sets of co-ordinates would appear to be the old radionic rates in a new and vastly more accurate form and *frame of reference*.

But Malcolm Rae has gone further and has investigated how this whole process appears to work in a human being.

We are born according to him, and I quote: "With an enormous number of sets of co-ordinates related to the many requirements of living on this planet, and we add to them subsequently by the experience of living." These co-ordinates can be activated when conscious *attention* is focussed on them, but — and I quote:

"Conscious mentation could not compute the required combinations of co-ordinates (and thus relative intensities) rapidly enough to sustain life in an environment which is liable to almost instantaneous change; and whatever it is in the subconscious that serves this purpose, in combination with the sets of co-ordinates available to it, is plainly able to achieve feats of mathematics which would confound our most sophisticated computers tended by their most competent programmers. Radiesthetic Q & A yielded, firstly that that which is responsible for energizing the appropriate co-ordinates to sustain life within those changes of environment which man was designed to withstand, is a Principle; and secondly, that the most accurate verbal description of it is 'the Essential Simplicity'."

and he comments:

"What an inspiring description that is too — the essential simplicity — the simplest and thus the most efficient employment of man's essence in conducting the behaviour of his substance!"

These two, i.e. "Attention" in the conscious and "Essential Simplicity" in the subconscious as designed by the Creator, should work perfectly together in harmony but since we are human beings we are constantly interfering and upsetting the programming. "The attempts of the 'essential simplicity' to cause the individual to take such steps as are required for bodily well-being, and to avoid those that are detrimental to it — culminate in complexities of compensation dis-intergative to the wholeness of the man."

In the light of all this, "therapy" becomes clear, and I quote: "In men, a boundary which has become a barrier, once it is correctly measured, may be treated with the appropriate corrective message in the form of a remedial pattern carried by an oral remedy or projected from a suitable instrument." This is where homoeopathy with its potentization comes into its own, as it provides the correct theraputic patterns which are necessary to once more restore wholeness.

This is only the barest, and, I fear, inadequate outline of this important paper, which of course contains more than I have mentioned, so it should be read in full, as these results of years of research work, appear to be basic truths as measured by the truth chart. There is a part of a prayer by Thomas Aquinas which runs like this: "Grant me penetration to understand, capacity to retain, method and facility in study, subtlety in interpretation and abundant grace of expression" which expresses what Rudolf Steiner saw as necessary to modern times and I quote: that ". . . it is not by mystical experience which divorces itself from reason and despises logic, that man returns to his spiritual heritage, but by the path of pure, concentrated thinking in which logic is never contradicted."

Jane Wilcox and Malcolm Rae would not have arrived at these important discoveries and conclusions if they had not exercised increasingly clear, precise and exact thinking – the formulation of true thoughts – in all this Q & A work. Their aim was the pursuit of truth, and so they learnt to ask creatively for the truth and therefore received it, obeying the injunction "Ask and it shall be given unto you."

But there is still a difficulty.

On the title page of Part II of my book *Life Threatened*, I have this quotation:

"Two thousand years ago, Christ initiated human feeling and devotion into faith in the spirit-world and in the reality of man's spiritual destiny, and so made possible the evolution of his ego-consciousness and the development of his powers of thought. To-day He would make possible for him the recovery in clear knowledge and understanding of his true spirit-heritage, by initiating his thinking into direct spirit experience. The redemption of thinking is the completion of the spirit-initiation of mankind by Christ."

I put it there because I felt it to be profoundly true and of the greatest importance, yet I could not see that any but a very small minority could attain to sense-free thinking which was said to be requisite if this was to be done and which only adepts such as Steiner could accomplish. It seems to rule out the vast majority of us, bogged down as we are in our material values and ways of thought, and yet it seems essential we should try, so that we too could discover, to quote Steiner "that besides powers and possibilities of thinking as an instrument of knowledge it had functions of which man had lost all knowledge, viz., a creative function – that it operated as a creative formative force in the life of man both in the spiritual and physical world".

In meditating upon all this it came to me that perhaps in the technique of Q & A we had already been given an answer, that all who practise Q & A in spirit and in truth are in fact bringing about the redemption of thinking and recovering its lost creative functions, with all the incredible consequences for good that would ensue, such as the complete transformation of science so that it becomes "a science of Reality, which would embrace both material science and spiritual science in one majestic whole – a true science of the cosmos".

So maybe in the end the ultimate role and scope of the radiesthetic faculty in the modern world is the redemption of thinking – a bridge between two worlds.

Let me end with this quotation from my book the *Pattern of Health* written in 1961 in which I appear to have foretold the role and scope of the radiesthetic faculty, as it had unfolded in the last 11 years:

"All human thinking, since the Fall of Man, is liable to error and untruth, only through the Spirit of Truth can we be preserved in this materialistic age from falsehood and destructive thinking. I believe it is literally true, insofar as science is the search for truth, that Christ — the Way, the Truth and the Life — is a scientific necessity, and this applies equally, strange as it may seem, to such a humble science as Radiesthesia.

"'God hath chosen the foolish things of this world to confound the wise and God hath chosen the weak things of the world to confound the things that are mighty;

"'And base things of the world, and things which are despised, hath God chosen, yea, and things which are not, to bring to naught things that are.'

"In the eyes of the world Radiesthesia is a thing of no account compared with, say, nuclear or astro-physics or atomic research, and yet, as I have tried to show, it can, when properly understood, open to us the mysteries both in this world and the world invisible. It can reveal to us the Truth in so far as our finite minds can comprehend it.

"I believe profoundly that it is the privilege of Radiesthesia to make its very special and, in some ways, unique contribution to the reintegration of material science and spiritual science, and to that restoration of wholeness of vision and outlook, of feeling and thinking which is the task of this age."

At first glance material science and spiritual science may seem strange bed-fellows, but it is remarkable how esoteric knowledge can provide a deeper understanding of material factors. In a lecture given in the 1930's by Dr. Gladys Shutt, D.C. at Topeka, she spoke of how radionic broadcast treatments harmonized the vibratory rate of the various body tissues, and she goes on to pose the question:

How is this accounted for physiologically? As has been pointed out earlier, the energy which activates our tissues is in the nature of light; it has the speed and the qualities of light. A common experiment of the biology laboratory is that of sending a beam of light against a one-celled organism and noting the effect of that beam in intensifying the activity within the nucleus of the cell until cleavage of the cell nucleus finally takes place.

The application of this scientific fact answers the question as to what occurs under the Drown Method. We have a beam of light — a "radio beam" if you please — being sent into the tissue in the wavelength of that tissue itself. Through the process of metabolism and cell division constantly going on in the body, accentuated in the structure into which the body energy is being concentrated, the new cells will come in at a higher rate of vibration and the diseased cells will automatically fall away. Since like poles repel and unlike poles attract, cell division obviously takes place when the invisible light (positive in its polarity) strikes the positively charged nucleus of the cell. Abnormal disease vibration can no more continue to exist in normally vibrating tissue than light and darkness can exist in the same spot.

Here one point must be made clear. In diagnosing, we wish to receive the energy emanating from the disease formation itself, and we deal with that alone. In treating, however, the disease energy is not sent back into the part in its own vibration, even though the dial settings are the same as those found in diagnosis. Instead, the reception of the total body energy is localized through the treatment hook-up; the dial setting is a means of localizing the area into which the energy is being sent.

For instance, even though we find tuberculosis of the lung in diagnosis, and utilize that same dial setting for treatment, we are following a pattern, first, of localizing the energy reception in the lung by tuning into that lung, and second, of further localizing it by specifying the tubercular tissue of the lung for the reception of the energy wave-lengths which will cause stimulation and rehabilitation. We are not shattering the diseased tissue in a concentration of its own rate, but intensifying the rebuilding process of cell division in that particular area. Through this process, the normal will exclude the abnormal of its own accord, and a healthy state will be created.

These facts are scientific, acceptable, authoritative, backed by laboratory and clinical proof, and based on known experiments and conclusions.

Now from an orthodox standpoint Dr. Shutt's presentation and theory is probably full of holes. If however the practitioner is prepared to step beyond the borderlines of his 'medical posture' he will see that what she has to say opens other doors. As far as she is concerned her theory as presented above is proven by the weight of clinical evidence; people get well from treatment based on the premises which she has set forth. I would like, for just a moment to consider her use of the word light, which she uses to denote the healing energy projected in radionic treatment. Material science of course would want to set up devices and instrumentation to measure this 'light' and no doubt upon completion of their tests would say it does not exist; and for orthodoxy that would be the end of the matter. Light in spiritual science has other connotations and must be seen and measured through the sensitivity of the observing individual. Light in these terms is a subjective phenomena, yet every bit as real as electric light, if not more so. Curiously Dr. Shutt speaks of tuberculosis in almost the same breath as light, in her lecture. So What? you may think, but consider Steiner's thoughts on these factors, and see how doors open in spiritual science if you will allow them to:

But at the borderline between ourselves and the world outside, something very significant happens to light, that is, to something purely etheric; it becomes transmuted. And if needs must be transmuted. For, consider how the process of plant formation is held up in man, how this process is so to speak broken off and counteracted by the process that manufactures carbon dioxide. In the same way, the process contained in the life of light is interrupted in man. And so, if we seek for light within man, it must be something transformed, it must be a metamorphosis of light.

At the moment of crossing the borderline of man inwards, we find a metamorphosis of light. This means that man does not only transform the common, ponderable processes of external nature within himself, but also the imponderable element — Light itself. He changes it into something different. And if the bacillus of tuberculosis thrives in the human interior and perishes in the full sunlight, it is evident — to a sound judgement of the fact — that the product of the light as transmuted within us, must offer a favourable environment to these bacilli, and if they multiply excessively, there must be something wrong with the product of transmutation, and thence we get the insight that amongst the causes of tuberculosis is involved that of the process of transmutation of light within the patient. Something occurs which should not occur, otherwise he would not harbour too many of the tuberculosis bacilli — for they are always present in all of us, but as a rule in insufficient numbers to provoke active tuberculosis. If they are too prolific, their "host" succumbs to the disease. And the tuberculosis bacillus could not be found everywhere, if there were not something abnormal in the development of this transmuted light of the sun. . . .

What happens if a human being becomes suitable soil for tuberculosis bacilli that is either he is not constitutionally capable of absorbing sunlight, or he does not get enough sunlight to absorb, owing to his way of life. Thus there is not an adequate balance between the amount of sunlight he receives from outside, and the amount he can transmute; and this forces him to draw reserves from the already transmuted light stored up within him.

Please pay particular attention to this: Man, by the very fact of being man, has a continuous supply of stored and transmuted light within. That is necessary to his organisation. If the mutual process, enacted between man and the external sunlight, does not take place properly, his body is deprived of the transmuted light.

Other authors in the esoteric field write in the same vein as Steiner. For example Ethel Belle Morrow in her book *The One Universal Law* says:

> The great emanation of light from God, the Father, acts as the neutron of the universe; and the rays of light, contacting the forces, make the interchange, as reflection and absorption of the white light. The energy, stored, as the stabilization of the forces in both elements and plants, helps to rebuild the soma cells of man, but the contacts of unbalanced forces of the elements are seldom inert to admit the inflow of life. The process must need go through the procedure of the Law, that of balance in the elements for mineral which are used toward balance for plant life and balance in the plant towards balance in animals and man, before the One Power as spirit can become the life of the form. The energy of the sunlight, as an emanation from God, gives manifestation to all atomic forces, under the One Law.
>
> Man radiates colors as the manifestation of various positive and negative combinations of forces; these may be balanced into the white light of purity, through the quickening of the spirit.
>
> In the thought forces, the balance is quickly obtained through faith which permits, if man so wills, the entrance of the white light as spiritual mind power. This, as spiritual consciousness, allows the life to be retained in the blood. Man's organisms, without his white light as power, become a slime-mould of darkness.
>
> Love is the dynamic force which tends to keep the white light in evidence; for love is the drawing power of God which connects the individual to the Universal Mind of God, as spiritual consciousness.

In *The Theory and Technique of the Drown Radio-Therapy and Radio-Vision Instruments* Ruth Drown frequently refers to the Radiant Energy of the body. She writes:

> This is the Energy that creates individuals in all phases of life, and it is the amount of Life Force (which is an invisible light, passing through the brain, the nervous system and the blood vessels) which animates all these bodies, making one human being healthy, and another, through its lack, in a state of dis-ease.

The concept of the energy which vitalises the human form as light, may at first be difficult to come to terms with. But as Drown points out, the light can be used to bring harmony through radionic therapy, to the cellular structures of the body. Her radionic photographs of the etheric counterparts of organs and tissues, taken in total darkness, substantiate her theories beyond any argument. Light in the form of the universal Life Force sweeping across the emulsion of the film, leaves images of striking clarity, in which raised areas literally throw shadows. A series of these etheric photographs taken by Drown appear in my other book 'Interface' and they are well worth studying relative to this concept of light.

Radionics, as an approach to healing has been sustained and kept alive by the lay-practitioner for many years now, without them it may well have perished, instead it has gone from strength to strength evolving and developing to the point where once again health-care professionals from various disciplines are taking a keen interest in it. Radionics has much to offer any doctor, chiropractor or osteopath who is prepared to cross the interfaces between disciplines and widen his horizons. How the individual practitioner will be able to make use of radionics in his practice will naturally depend on many factors, but even the analysis of difficult cases alone has much to commend it. The selection of drugs, homoeopathic remedies or other treatments and the accurate determination of strength and dosage through the use of the radiesthetic faculty can prove to be a boon in any practice. Probably for all practitioners the use of individual radionic treatments is a time consuming stumbling block, which can be overcome of course if one has an assistant that deals with this end of the practice under the watchful eye of the doctor. The use of an automatic treatment device with a Comprehensive Therapy Radio card (see *Radionics Interface with the Ether Fields*) may also be employed in order to cut out having to deal with each patient one at a time. From my own experience I would say that if the practitioner intends to make any kind of extensive use of radionics along with his own practice, he will almost certainly need an assistant. Dealing with a radionic patient is not like dealing with a patient, say for manipulation of the spine where the treatment is given and then they leave. Radionic patients are always with you, and you are as close to them as the telephone, which some make more than good use of for every little emergency.

Magneto-Geometric potency simulation and the Potency Preparer can be used extensively in any practice where remedies are used, and they are time saving, effective and proven in the field by numerous medical doctors. This is an aspect of radionics, which I have said before, may appeal to the doctor who is still doubtful in his mind about the practical realities of diagnosis and treatment at a distance, but is prepared to use the Simulator or the Preparer on the basis of their proven effectiveness.

Whoever takes up radionics is embarking on a journey that will lead him or her from the world of physical form to the realities beyond, and ultimately to the practice of true spiritual healing. The practice of radionics hones, sharpens and prepares the mind in ways that will make it a clear channel for the energies of the soul, and although radionics is primarily a mental approach to healing, the soul of the practitioner is inevitably involved to a greater or lesser degree in the process. In *Esoteric Healing* Alice Bailey lists a series of points which should be understood by anyone who seeks to heal, and this most definitely includes radionic practitioners.

It will be obvious that the healer, as he trains himself in the healing art, has to grasp clearly and candidly certain exceedingly simple yet esoteric facts:

1. That healing is simply and essentially the manipulation of energies.
2. That he must carefully differentiate between energies and forces.
3. That if he seeks real success, he must learn to place the patient as accurately as possible upon the correct rung of the ladder of evolution.
4. That knowledge of the centres is imperative.
5. That he himself must work as a soul through his personality.
6. That his relation to the patient (unless the latter is highly evolved) is a personality one.
7. That he must locate the centre controlling the area which involves the point of friction.
8. That, as with all else in the occult sciences, disease and healing are both aspects of the great "relationship" system which governs all manifestation.

If the healer will take these eight points and reflect and brood upon them, he will lay a sound foundation for all work to be done, their relative simplicity is such that it will be obvious that anyone can be a healer if he so chooses and he is willing to conform to the requirements. The current idea that a person is a "born" healer, and therefore unique, in reality indicates only that it is one of his main directed interests. Therefore, because of this interest, his attention has been turned towards the healing art and consequently towards contact with patients; owing to the inevitable working of the law which governs thought, he discovers that energy follows his thought and flows through him to the patient. When he does this with deliberation, a healing will often follow. Any man or woman — given real interest and prompted by the incentive to serve — who thinks and loves, can be a healer, and it is time people grasped that fact. The entire process of healing is thought-directed; it concerns the direction of energy currents or their abstraction, and this is another way of speaking about radiation and magnetism.

The above passages have much in them that will be of use to radionic practitioners, and they provide an overall guide as to some of the basic factors which must be taken into consideration by anyone who wants to work effectively in this field.

Radionics has within it the seeds of a new medicine, and it is hoped that this book will serve to stimulate health-care professionals to look further into this subject, and to consider how they may be able to benefit their patients through the use of radionic techniques. It is hoped too, that what has been written will encourage many young aspiring lay-practitioners to 'render themselves effective' in such a way that they will have no difficulty in taking up radionics as a full-time healing profession, and to build their own practices or find places as assistants to practitioners in other disciplines. There is, I am sure, a wide untapped field of service here for many young people with their gifts of sensitivity and healing.

With the growing experimentation in the field of Magneto-Biology, the use of Kirlian photography for diagnostic purposes, and the extensive research into action and influence at a distance, the stage is being set for science to make its entry into an era of etheric investigation. The bridge between the physical and subtle worlds has been intuited and sensed by many, now the means by which the invisible can be made visible will emerge. Radionics began with Abrams during the last quarter of the nineteenth century, who came, as I have mentioned elsewhere with a host of other 'light bearers' such as Roentgen, the Curies, Tesla and the Impressionist painters. Once again the surging flow of the evolutionary forces is bringing a new wave of light as we enter the last quarter of the twentieth century. What new discoveries this will bring, who the new 'light bearers' are, remains to be seen. One thing is certain however, Abrams planted the seed which has been nurtured for less than seventy years, and now radionics is about to burst forth and be transformed into a healing art beyond our imagination.

POTENCY CALCULATION GRAPHS FOR USE WITH
THE EXTENDED RANGE POTENCY SIMULATOR

GRAPH A

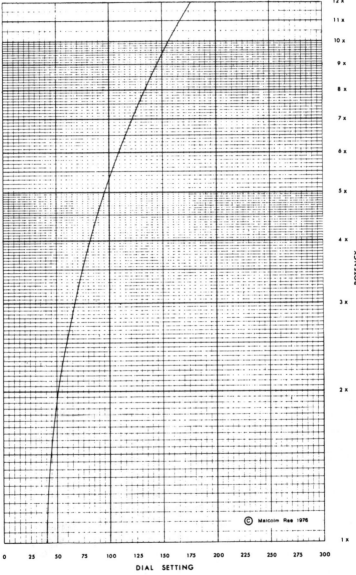

RAE EXTENDED RANGE POTENCY SIMULATOR – SETTING CHART

GRAPH B

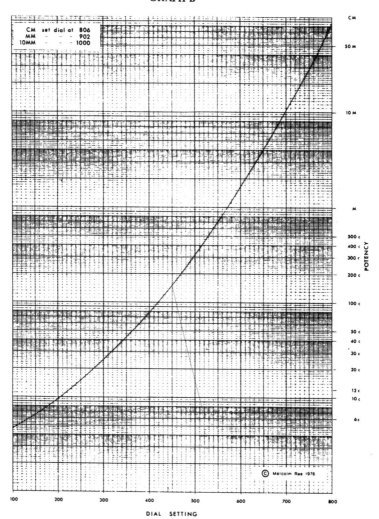

RAE EXTENDED RANGE POTENCY SIMULATOR – SETTING CHART

Enquiries about the Rae Magneto-Geometric Radionic Analyser, the Mark III Potency Simulator, the Extended Range Simulator, the Multiple Remedy Potency Simulator and the Potency Preparer should be addressed to:

Magneto-Geometric Applications
45 Downhill Road
London SE6 15X
England

The above listed instruments are available only to those having recognised qualifications in a recognised therapeutic discipline. All enquiries should be accompanied by a stamped addressed envelope, or if coming from abroad, by an International Reply Coupon.

For general information about radionics enquiries should be addressed to:

The Secretary,
The Radionics Association
Baerlein House, Goose Green
Deddington
Banbury
Oxon OX15 0SZ
England

Or:

The Radionic Magnetic Centre Organisation,
De La Warr Laboratories Ltd.,
Raleigh Park Road,
Oxford OX2 9BB,
Oxon.

DAVID V. TANSLEY BIBLIOGRAPHY

Subtle Body– Essence and Shadow, Thames & Hudson
The Raiment of Light, A Study of the Human Aura, Arkana Books
Omens of Awareness, Neville Spearman Ltd.
Radionics and the Subtle Anatomy of Man, The C.W. Daniel Company
Radionics—Interface with the Ether Fields, The C.W. Daniel Company
Radionics: Science or Magic?, The C.W. Daniel Company
Radionics– A Patient's Guide, Element Books
Chakras—Rays and Radionics, The C.W. Daniel Company
Ray Paths and Chakra Gateways, The C.W. Daniel Company

OTHER TITLES OF INTEREST FROM BROTHERHOOD OF LIFE

Rhythm & Touch, An Introduction to Craniosacral Therapy,
          Anthony P. Arnold
Shamanic Healing within The Medicine Wheel, Marie-Lu Lörler
The Spirits' Book, Allan Kardec
Prodigal Genius, The Life of Nikola Tesla, John J. O'Neill
The Lost Continent of Mu series by Col. James Churchward
The Aghora series by Robert E. Svoboda
Yoga Sutras of Patanjali, Charles Johnston translation
          and many others
          Titles List Available Upon Request

Distributed in the U.K. by
The C.W. Daniel Company Ltd.
1 Church Path
Saffron Walden
ESSEX CB10 1JP